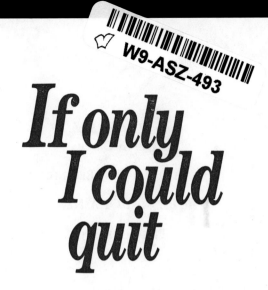

If only I could quit

RECOVERING FROM NICOTINE ADDICTION

Other Hazelden Books by
Karen Casey

EACH DAY A NEW BEGINNING

THE PROMISE OF A NEW DAY

THE LOVE BOOK

If only I could quit

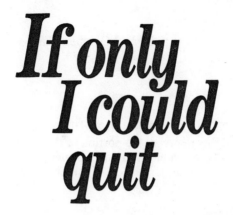

RECOVERING FROM NICOTINE ADDICTION

Karen Casey

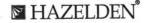

HAZELDEN®

First published October, 1987.

ISBN: 0-89486-438-6

Library of Congress Catalog Number:
87-80030

Printed in the United States of America.

CONTENTS

PERSONAL STORIES

MEDITATIONS

AFTERWORD

INDEX

ACKNOWLEDGMENTS

I learned so much from writing this book. In its own way, each story I listened to helped me better understand my own personal commitment to being a nonsmoker. I deeply thank each man and woman who took the time to talk with me. It's my hope that I've conveyed their stories accurately, without distortion, and with a sense of their love for all who want to join our ranks as nonsmokers.

I especially want to thank my husband, Joe, for exploring with me the direction this book should take. Initially I was off course and he risked sharing his perception and, in the process, guided me to the book's present form. His instincts were wonderful and on target. I loved our collaboration.

And I want to thank you, the reader, for daring to risk living life free of tobacco. The road will feel long and lonely at times, but there are millions of us who have gone before and our spirits are traveling with you. As our numbers multiply, our environment grows safer for all humanity. Future generations will reap many blessings from our courageous decision. Peace be with you.

INTRODUCTION

My Story

The refrigerator still held its accustomed two-carton stock of cigarettes that cold December evening, just five days short of Christmas, when events mysteriously paved the way for my becoming a nonsmoker. Members of my women's A.A. group had gathered at my apartment to bring the program to me because I had been ill and was unable to get to them.

As we sat around the Christmas tree in my tiny living room, Rita began talking about her desire to quit smoking. She wanted to make that her gift to her family on that Christmas in 1976. Although the topic wasn't A.A., it was quickly apparent that it was a First Step issue. Rita was not the only one among us addicted to nicotine, and we easily saw the parallels between our struggles with alcohol and other drugs and the current struggle with cigarettes. It was true, all of our lives were controlled by our need to smoke wherever and whenever we could.

I was personally startled when I enumerated the activities that "demanded" I smoke. Driving, talking with a friend, coffee, awaiting dinner (or lunch or breakfast) in a restaurant (or at home), phone conversations, or waiting on a call, leisure bathing in a tub, the morning alarm, the many visits to the bathroom throughout the day, reading a good or a bad book for pleasure or a class, writing a letter, or a grocery list or a paper for one of my graduate courses, hurt feelings, anger,

3

fear of abandonment, an actual or an imagined confrontation with a friend or lover, applying makeup, drying my hair, dressing for the day or evening, unwinding, preparing for bed, visiting with my Higher Power before turning out the light, cleaning house, outlining the day's activities, daydreaming, and obsessive thinking about my life or "him" or "what if." The list was endless. I was embarrassed, but I loved smoking. I felt supportive of Rita's desire to quit, but I was quite content to carry on as usual. When friends were in need, however, I was quick to offer an ear, and sometimes unwanted advice.

The next thing I knew the words came tumbling out. But they weren't musts and shoulds; rather, they were gentle suggestions coming from some place deep within me. I heard myself speaking, but I wasn't sure who was formulating the ideas I was mouthing. "Why not make a decision to be a nonsmoker, Rita? A nonsmoker doesn't grab for her cigarettes and lighter when the phone rings. A nonsmoker can even go to the bathroom empty-handed or choose to go out for the evening purseless or matchless! A nonsmoker is free to make new choices about places to visit or activities to participate in because the first allegiance is to oneself — not to a pack of cigarettes."

I truly didn't know where my message was coming from. I was simply the messenger, a steadily puffing messenger at that. "Rita," I said, "the desire for a cigarette doesn't even cross a nonsmoker's mind. This person is free to focus on

4

an engaging conversation, the chirping birds outside the open window, and the laughter of the children on the stairs. There is no resentment about not being able to smoke because one's identity is as a nonsmoker." I knew that plain and simply, a nonsmoker isn't haunted by the urge to inhale the taste of tobacco.

But I was just as certain at that moment that when a smoker quit, he or she felt deprived; after all, cigarettes were friends who comforted. Cigarettes brought relief. It was no wonder I felt this way. A decade earlier, in 1966, I had tried to quit smoking. I had not, however, changed my self-perception. Although I did not smoke for six years, I was, at heart, still a smoker who (damn it!) didn't smoke anymore. What a relief when I finally let go of my control over it and took the plunge back into the haven of "cigaretteville." When I resumed smoking, it was with a vengeance. I was making up for lost time; it seemed almost based on anger. My consumption quickly escalated from one pack to nearly three packs daily. And never did I think of quitting again.

Yet, here I was, sharing a bit of inner wisdom with Rita about the positive aspects of smoking no more. The subtle difference between quitting a loved addiction and becoming a new personality was not lost on me, however! Moments later my speech ended and so did that phase of my personal history. I very quietly put out my cigarette and have been a nonsmoker ever since.

I can't say that my physical body was as content with the new self-perception as was my mind. My body cried out for nicotine — loudly at times. I had heard that smoking muffled our feelings, but I didn't know how much. And I was to know a new level of rage. On not-too-rare occasions in the first three months after I had quit, all 115 pounds of me startled others as well as myself when, with contempt, I screamed at unsuspecting people who wandered across my path. "What do you mean I need to tell you what weight oil to put in my car! You work here, don't you?"

But my self-talk saved me. At frequent intervals throughout each morning, each afternoon, and each evening, I took a few moments "away" from the people or task at hand to image myself as a smiling, confident nonsmoker. Fortunately, I also had a Higher Power and a Twelve Step program for strength. I was soon to discover, however, there wasn't great support from many of my friends and acquaintances in school, at work, or at my meetings. But the strength to continue on was sustained. And with each passing day, I more firmly filled the body and the shoes of my nonsmoking self.

I detected a healthy ego response, too. It exhilarated me that I had reclaimed some personal power over my identity. I had chosen a new posture toward life; I had chosen to quit killing myself, a puff at a time. The natural deduction was that I was learning to love myself — a first step to loving someone else. When the old Karen tugged at me to return to the old ways — and she did, frequently at first but with lessening frequency as time elapsed — the new me was able to stand my ground. I was a nonsmoker and so proud of it. I was free to sit where I wanted in restaurants. My hair and clothes no longer reeked of tobacco. My apartment didn't smell like a crowded bar any longer. And after washing my car and apartment windows, I was treated to a new brightness wherever I looked. With disgust, I wiped away the yellow nicotine stains from the glass protecting the many pictures hung throughout my apartment, and my commitment to my nonsmoking life was strengthened.

Who would have thought back in 1955 that this choice would capture me in 1976? I thought smoking was sexy then. I remember all too well riding down 9th Street with Barbara in her mother's white two-door Chevy. Barbara needed both hands to steer and shift the car so the cigarette dangled from her lips. I took one from the red and white box-top pack and waited for the cigarette lighter to pop out. My ears buzzed with the first deep draw and my head felt light. But we giggled, feeling so smart and sophisticated. My first cigarette had been at a slumber party in ninth grade. But that was just girl stuff and no inhaling. This was different. This was the real thing. We had a car, a half tank of gas, and a full pack of Marlboros between us on the seat and the evening was young.

It was understood in my family that I'd be a smoker. They were all smokers, parents, aunts and uncles, grandparents, even my two older sisters. My dad requested that I not smoke until the age of eighteen, so I dutifully lied about it and hid my smoking; then, on my eighteenth birthday, I was given a carton of cigarettes as a present. It was my passage to adulthood.

And here I was, 21 years later saying, "Wait a minute, I want to make a new choice; to have a new identity." And so close on the heels of my turn to A.A., too. A fortunate, life-giving choice it was. The rewards have been many. I wish I could say Rita remained a nonsmoker as well. But after a few months, she returned to smoking. She was there for me through my trying times, though, and the phone lines between our homes buzzed with affirmations, cries for help, and prayers.

With confidence and full certainty, readers, I can assure you that my life as a nonsmoker is rewarding. There is no doubt that I'm healthier. My energy level is higher. I accomplish more daily because I'm not taking the accustomed cigarette breaks of years past. I play better racquetball and tennis. Hurrying up steps doesn't wind me. My hair, breath, clothes, and home no longer smell like a barroom floor. My teeth no longer have brown stains. My fingertips are a healthy pink. And I haven't lost my desire or ability to write. How certain I was that writing and cigarettes were tightly entwined. My fear was great that nonsmoking Karen would also be nonwriting Karen. However, I have four books under my belt as proof that whatever wisdom I've been blessed with to share, it didn't come from cigarettes.

What follows next are stories of other "recovering" smokers. There is so much each of us can gain from helping and being helped by "one who has gone before." Please read on — for the strength, the hope, and the courage to quit. Another benefit of the stories is the realization that's sure to come to you that we're all so very much alike, even though the details of our lives may differ. Giving up tobacco is a major decision. It was for each of us. But it's one worth making. Together we can accomplish the task.

MARY

Age 33. Married, completing an M.A. in adult education; employed as a staff trainer in a Fortune 500 company; loves reading, skiing, working out, and cats; she's great at writing and making others laugh.

I remember so vividly when I started smoking. I have blurred memories about lots of my life, but my smoking history stands out real clearly. I was in sixth grade when a lot of my friends started smoking. At the beach, my best friend and I decided we weren't going to smoke. We thought it was real slutty and we were not going to be sluts.

Next thing I remember is three years later and we're in my friend Terri's basement. I'm a freshman in high school. I had made it through seventh and eighth grade and actually had no desire to smoke and thought it looked stupid. I hated to see girls on the street smoking. So here we are sitting around Terri's piano; we have a pack of Old Golds, and we're learning to smoke. Her parents are out of town and we're highly motivated to learn. I don't know what changed in those three years other than I began to identify myself more with grown ups. Smoking took on more glamour. It was no longer street tough. By now all the girls I knew at school, who were older, smoked. It became for me a rite of passage. We all got very sick that first time on the pack of Old Golds, but we sort of knew that that was part of the process and we'd soon get over it.

I have some other early memories related to smoking. My friend, Terri, lived three houses away from me and we used to walk back and forth between our houses. On one school night in late fall we were outside in the back alley and four or five of us were smoking. We were still really new at it and it was a very conscious act. After that, I was a smoker and wanted to be a smoker. All but one of my sisters smoked too, as did all my friends at school. That first year I lost fifteen pounds. From then on, smoking was a very deliberate way of weight control. I didn't sit around and think Gee, if I smoke I won't get fat. But somehow I knew that I had replaced a lot of my eating behavior with cigarettes. I got an immediate payoff.

In high school, we smoked in the bathrooms all the time. We passed those hot butts around. We could hardly hold on to them, they were so hot. Everybody knew we were smoking but they didn't put much pressure on us to quit. They could have clamped down much harder, but they chose to ignore it.

I smoked all through high school and really got a lot of pleasure from being one of the crowd. When I got out of high school, I did a lot of drugs and alcohol, and smoking became a part of me. It became a part of my identity. I was a heavy smoker and I felt more confident when I was with a cigarette than when I was not with a cigarette. I loved smoking, for the fifteen years I smoked.

11

I felt really powerful when I smoked, and the cigarette was sort of an extension of my mystique. I always had friends who smoked too. I didn't know people who were nonsmokers; I was not attracted to them. Smokers were the big part of my social network. Now that I think back, I did have one good friend who didn't smoke — Jimmy, who was crazy, wild, and wonderful. We ran around and did a lot of drugs and a lot of partying. He was a real funny, funny guy and he never smoked. He always used to rag about people who smoked. He thought it was obnoxious, ugly, terrible, and unhealthy, but he was really in the minority. I can remember being amazed that he didn't smoke and surprised that he was so offended by it.

For years I smoked with intent even though in the seventies nonsmoking was becoming popular. I made a conscious decision that I was not going to stop smoking because I had just stopped drinking. I got support from people who reinforced the notion that you shouldn't quit everything at once. I lived in a halfway house with 30 women, and 29 of us smoked. The poor woman who didn't smoke was in a cloud of smoke all the time and we just beat her up about it. "What do you mean you don't want us to smoke at the dinner table?" When I was in therapy, everybody smoked and it was great. It was something to focus on when everything was going awry. I smoked heavier after I quit drinking than at any other time in my life. I did more morning smoking.

I just loved cigarettes when I was in college and studying for exams because I would get up in the morning as early as three o'clock, make a pot of coffee and sit down when it was perfectly quiet. I had a pack of cigarettes and my books and I would study, smoke, and drink coffee until nine or ten o'clock. It was almost spiritual. From that early morning smoking, I'd get a real chemical high. The early morning seemed to always be the time when the cigarettes and the coffee worked the best. I didn't like going to the library because I couldn't smoke there. I used to carry all these books around with me and go home where I could smoke and study.

About a year ago, I read some results of a study that concluded that nicotine had an effect on the brain that caused increased concentration. I knew it was true for me. The hardest thing for me when I was trying to make a decision to quit was that internal knowledge that smoking was a stimulus that was helpful to me. And I had said to myself, "I am going to smoke until I'm 30." And that was when I was 22. Whenever the subject came up, I said, "I'm not even going to consider quitting until I'm 30." And then I smoked in total enjoyment and lack of guilt for eight years. I smoked my guts out. As I approached 30, I got real nervous. But by then I started to have some consequences from smoking.

One night I had stayed up writing something and I got so excited about what I was writing that I didn't want to go to bed. I stayed up and smoked and smoked. I slept maybe two hours that night. I was so excited about what I was working on that I got right up in the morning, put on a pot of coffee and sat down to work with a cigarette, but I could hardly inhale. My chest hurt so badly. I noticed that often my chest ached and I had to back off from smoking in the morning.

Gradually I started to open myself up to information about the harmful effects of smoking. I'd really cut myself off from that information. I didn't want to hear it. I had never thought about it. As I approached 30 and was having some consequences, I started considering a little more openly why smoking really was bad. I read a couple articles that blew my mind. I always worried about quitting because I always worried about gaining weight. That entire eight-year period when I smoked so heavily, I used it very deliberately for weight control. I wasn't working out and I wasn't taking care of myself. I was having a lot of conflict as I approached the goal to quit. I had a lot invested in smoking. I was just starting graduate school. And yet, I was also starting to realize how bad smoking was for me. Many heavy smokers I knew were quitting and I was curious about that. I was hearing their quitting stories, and I was beginning to feel peer pressure. I didn't want to get left in the smoke. Smoking was getting more unfashionable and I was getting more self-conscious.

The first time I quit smoking was after another night when I had been up late reading, writing, and smoking. I got up early in the morning and had a bad cigarette hangover. I sat down, opened up the morning paper and read an article about how the tobacco industry was beside itself that so many people were quitting smoking. They had come up with this new marketing strategy. They were going into third world countries and selling cigarettes at a very reduced cost and getting people hooked on them. I read the article and I was appalled. I was just so sickened because I was a smoker and I was supporting that. Every time I lit up I was encouraging or participating in the complete annihilation of human health. I quit smoking that day. I could not pick up a cigarette all day; I was just sickened by that article. I stayed off cigarettes for three months that first time. And that surprised me.

Right after I quit, my husband and I joined a health club. That was my reward. I was so out of shape that I was not able to swim two laps. I remember the first week I quit; I was in an all-week workshop for graduate school. I was so out of touch because of withdrawal. I can remember listening to the instructor, having his words kind of come at me and go away, come at me and go away. That whole week I was so exhausted I'd go to bed right after I got home and sleep all night. I couldn't keep my eyes open.

What kept me from smoking was pride, just pride. I wasn't comfortable and I wasn't enjoying it. I was really preoccupied with smoking. I was proving to myself I could do it. That was what kept me going those first three months. I cried all the time. I was real vulnerable those first six weeks and overly sensitive. I felt exposed when I was with people. But I knew it was withdrawal. My husband quit at the same time and we would argue about any little thing. For about six weeks we were rageful. It calmed down towards the end of the summer, but then on a trip to Montreal I started smoking. I was fed up with being preoccupied about not smoking. It hadn't gone away. It was there, and it was minute-to-minute. It felt like it was getting worse instead of getting better. I can remember, on the way to Montreal, going into a drugstore for cigarettes. Buying them was an escape out of this madness. I was uncomfortable. I was unhappy. I was rageful. I was not myself, and I was no longer glamorous. I felt odd and I felt disoriented. I knew all I had to do was buy a pack of cigarettes and it would all go away. And it did. That was the scariest part. Within ten cigarettes, I was back into a complete, secure identity.

I felt so guilty. I never told my husband until after I had smoked a pack of cigarettes. I was really concerned about how I was going to tell him. So I figured I would quit again. Either that or go to the bathroom a lot because we were on our way to Montreal.

Four or five days into the trip, he started too. And then we had a wonderful time. We just smoked our way through Montreal. Things were just as hunky-dory as they'd always been. Then we tried to quit again on the way home. We were on this marathon drive back. We were going to do 1600 miles in a straight shot. On the first day,

16

we decided to quit. Eight hours later in this thrashing rainstorm in this little tiny car at 2:00 A.M. we started raging at each other. By the time we got to Chicago, we were smoking again.

I smoked for another year and then quit again after my husband's dad got cancer. My husband had quit immediately after he got the phone call about the cancer; he was through with smoking. I said right then and there, "I'm going to quit too, but I'm not going to do it right now." I felt like we shouldn't try to do it together. So three months later I finally quit. One morning I woke up with an incredible cigarette hangover and I said, "That's it. I'm done." It was a lot easier because I stayed off of sugar those first two months also. The withdrawal was 100 percent less intense for me when I was not doing sugar too. I was real surprised by how well I could manage the withdrawal. It would come and I could trust it would go away. To know that it wasn't going to go on every day made managing it possible. I remember, during that period, eating cake one night. I got crazy with nicotine withdrawal after I ate the piece of cake. It was clear to me that the two were connected.

After about three months, I noticed that I hadn't thought about smoking. I felt liberated by that. I was much more ready to quit. I was focusing on the little bits of relief from the obsession of smoking that were actually starting to come, and I built on them. I remember the first time I was with someone who smoked and I didn't want one. I started noticing I was changing. I felt so liberated that I was becoming a nonsmoker, and that I was released from the obsession. But this release didn't come until the third month. What was different this time was that I believed it would.

I got into aerobics. I had started working out when I'd quit before and I'd maintained a lot of my commitment to exercise during that time. Working out provided me with much physical relief. I had moments of serenity following a good aerobic workout which gave me a lot of strength and a lot of hope. With this quitting, I realized that I really was powerless and I trusted that if other people could do it, so could I. They served as my Higher Power.

I had about eight months of really good cigarette-free time, and then I started picking up cigarettes and smoking them. It only happened when I was with someone who was smoking. For six or eight months I'd have an occasional cigarette. At about this time my sister, who smoked, moved in with us temporarily. I made a deliberate decision that I was never going to smoke with her. She only smoked on the porch, not in the house. Never did I bum cigarettes from her. I did bum from others on probably sixteen different occasions in a six-month period. But I didn't want to be a smoker. The motivation not to be one was enough to keep me from falling completely back into it after I'd been in those situations. But when I would do it, I'd be having fun and I would remember how much more fun it was for me to smoke. I would just pick up a cigarette and smoke it compulsively. And I would sidestep any decision to quit. I smoked on Christmas day with my mother-in-law. She and I used to smoke together all the time. She was sharing some of her feelings and I was listening. I picked up one of her cigarettes and smoked it. I got so sick from the cigarette that I had to struggle to stay in the conversation. I had four puffs and put it out. That was the last time I smoked. I do have an incredible history with cigarettes. I have fantasies of smoking. I think my struggle will be life-long.

It seems hard for me to think that I would act compulsively and smoke again because I have so much shame. There'd be nowhere in my house that I could smoke without my husband having a fit. And I know so much about my health that I don't really think that I could do it.

I believe that I'll start to enjoy the writing process without smoking and that's what I'm going to have to focus on. I'll look for smaller rewards, like writing a page or two, and then taking a break or eating an orange or something. I'll do some behavior modification.

For the last three years, I've never smoked a cigarette on my job, never. I sit and write and concentrate and plan and do all sorts of activities at work and I don't have any problem not smoking. Even if somebody brought me a pack of cigarettes and said the surgeon general just changed his mind, I wouldn't pick one up at work. And I have found out that writing and not smoking has improved my concentration. I'm no longer getting wired. I may not start out as strong but I have much more stamina to concentrate. I'm less edgy and less frustrated, and I'm more effective.

I've learned through all of my false starts that coming to terms with being a nonsmoker is really coming to terms with taking responsibility for my health and changing my identity. I had to stop and start again but I was able to build on those experiences the next time. I needed to test the waters as I went along and I gained confidence in the process. It was just a matter of sticking to my decision and learning about it as I went and what to expect. Nonsmoking is so day-to-day. It's sometimes a minute-to-minute kind of new identity. Not every person is going to be successful on the first attempt. I certainly learned that giving up sugar for six weeks reduced the nicotine withdrawal. I also learned that contact with other people, trusting other people's experiences, and listening to other people's smoking stories helped me. When I was quitting, I felt it wasn't as intensive for others when they'd quit. It seemed others were always just sitting around drinking coffee and being casual about it. I had this sense that they were probably smokers who give up now and again and that they weren't really heavy smokers anyway.

The best thing about not smoking is that I did it. It doesn't have any power over me anymore. I think there were a lot of people who would have bet that I'd go back. I had that hard-core smoker image and many friends thought I'd still be tapping a cigarette on an ashtray at 70. A real plus of not smoking is that I can go out and run for a mile if I have to. I can go to an aerobics class and not even be hurting. When I was struggling with quitting, there were days that one of my motivations for not having a cigarette was that I couldn't workout and smoke, and I loved working out. I loved doing it so much that it helped me not to smoke.

Another benefit of not smoking is that I love being somewhere and not having to worry about it. Every time I see a smoker struggling with where and how to smoke, I'm so glad that it's not me. No longer am I struggling for an ashtray and an out-of-the-way place to smoke. It just gives me joy that I'm free. The hardest part for me has been gaining weight. I have gained fifteen pounds, the same fifteen pounds I lost when I started smoking.

It was very upsetting in the beginning, but I had to make a decision about my priorities. Once I made that decision, I was able to look at the weight gain as a part of my smoking problem. I look at compulsive behavior like this and I keep pulling the stops out. I'm determined not to worry about it, although some days I feel frantic. I have compulsive eating habits that didn't make sense before. I didn't see them because cigarettes broke the compulsive eating habit. I never saw myself out of control over food, but I was, so I joined Overeaters Anonymous. I see it as really related to my smoking. And I'm finding relief and a spiritual direction. This time I don't want to go back.

JIM

Age 82. Retired banker; happily married, father of four; hobbies are auto travel, bird-watching, and lawn care; avid basketball and football fan who loves dancing to the big band sounds of the thirties and forties.

I graduated from high school when I was seventeen years old, and when I was eighteen I left home and went to Logansport, Indiana and got a job as a brakeman on a railroad. That was in 1922. My dad smoked as far back as I can remember, but I was in Logansport for two or three years before I started to smoke, and really only began because everybody else my age was smoking cigarettes. It wasn't too long before I started to inhale.

When I was out on the railroad, I smoked a cob pipe rather than cigarettes. I'll never forget one time when I was going between Moran and Sedalia. I was riding on top of a boxcar on a local freight train that delivered groceries, cartons, cans, and boxes of bread. The locals were only eight, ten, or twelve cars long, and they stopped often, so in the summertime, instead of getting in the engine or caboose to ride from one town to another, I crawled up on top of a boxcar and sat there smoking my cob pipe as we went from Moran to Sedalia. One time I noticed the smoke tasted awful hot. We always wore gloves but I took the pipe out of my mouth and discovered that the whole side of the pipe was on fire. So I

22

quit smoking a cob pipe. However, I didn't quit cigarettes. It was "manly" to smoke. Even though I wasn't a man yet, but a boy, when I smoked cigarettes I felt like a man. And I continued to smoke throughout my life, for more than 40 years with no problems.

Not until getting close to the time when I actually quit did smoking ever bother me. Although there was talk about lung cancer, I had no sign of any lung cancer. I did have a touch of emphysema, so the doctor said, "Why don't you quit while you're even?" because emphysema progressively gets worse.

Shortly thereafter, we were at Fort Wayne for my birthday, and we went out to this nightclub where there was a band that played mostly Glenn Miller music. We sat there and had a beer or a drink or something and I thought, boy, this is my birthday, this would be an awful good time to quit. I'll always remember it, although I don't remember the year.

Actually, I had quit once years before. I had kids going to college and I got to thinking about how much it was costing me to smoke and how much better use I could put the money to even though cigarettes weren't high-priced then. So I quit. I didn't smoke for a year. I chewed a package of gum every day for weeks, instead of putting cigarettes in my mouth. But I crawled the wall sometimes needing tobacco so bad I thought I couldn't live without it. But I did live and when an urge came, I'd bite it off. I knew I didn't want to smoke again. But, of course, that didn't last forever. After about a year, I did start again and I don't know why. I started and kept steadily smoking until the last time I quit on my 60th birthday.

Like before, I had urges to smoke often. I was real nervous at first. I needed to keep busy, to keep doing something. On maybe a half-a-dozen occasions, I picked up my wife's cigarette and took a puff, never inhaled, just a puff. I'd get a mouthful and blow it out right away and that was the extent of it. But I don't take puffs anymore, I haven't for years. But even now, when somebody smokes aromatic pipe tobacco, that sets me off something wonderful. I could just grab his pipe and start puffing, but I never have.

After quitting for a while I soon noticed that everything tasted better than it did before. I think that's because the taste buds clear off. But I've never overeaten from nonsmoking, ever. And I didn't put on more than two or three or four extra pounds.

I've felt really good about not smoking. I'm proud of myself that I was able to quit at age 60, after having smoked nearly 40 years, and actually defy the urge to smoke. I just showed cigarettes a thing or two! I wasn't going to smoke and I'm kind of proud of that.

I'm sure not smoking has contributed in a positive way to my long life. I'm 82 now, nearly 83. When I think back on it, many in my family smoked. My Uncle George always smoked; Uncle Raymond always smoked. My granddad on my dad's side never did because he was a very, very religious fella. He used to smoke when he was young, they told me, but from the time I knew him as a granddad, I never knew him to ever smoke. My dad smoked a pipe as I was growing up at home. Then it was during that time that cigarettes came out and they were handier, quicker. So Dad started to smoke Camels and he smoked them until he died. Even my great, great grandmother smoked. When I was three or four years old, Mom used to take us to see Great-grandma Schaeffer and she smoked a clay pipe. I used to think that was so funny to see her sitting there in her chair holding her pipe, smoking. She always held it.

I miss cigarettes, even now after all these years. But I'm too bullheaded to give in and smoke now — but not just because of my emphysema. I've made up my mind it's a dirty habit. I quit and that's that! I just don't intend to smoke ever again. I do know this: if you're intimate with someone who smokes and you kiss them, you can smell it every time.

I feel great satisfaction at having been able to kick the habit and I feel good about myself for being able to stay away from cigarettes for 22 years. I only wish I'd live long enough to match the years I smoked with that many nonsmoking years but I doubt that I have that many years left.

JUDY

Age 35. Published writer, editor, former attorney whose loves are a gardening newsletter she has launched, intimate times with friends, and home ownership.

My parents were both heavy smokers when I was growing up. I remember going on car trips and being sick to my stomach because they were smoking in the car. I remember begging them to open the windows. My early experience said smoking was sickening.

Gradually medical reports were published about how bad smoking was. My parents, both doctors, were reading these reports and they decided to quit. My mom quit first. My dad struggled with it but they both had quit by the time I was in high school. The fact that they had quit probably prompted me to decide I was going to smoke. Besides, I thought it looked cool.

I remember seeing Lauren Bacall and Bette Davis in the movies and they smoked. They looked tough and cool and I thought they were really neat. In general, it was cooler to smoke than not to smoke. I had a friend who never smoked simply because her mom was a real heavy chain-smoker. Her mom died while we were in high school. She had an operation for lung cancer and died right after the operation. But that experience didn't phase me. My grandfather died of emphysema and I knew that was connected to his smoking but that didn't phase me either. To me, at fifteen, smoking was cool.

I remember my first cigarette made me dizzy. I tried to smoke without coughing so no one would know it was my first one. I was at our cabin. All of us kids snuck away to try cigarettes. I practiced a lot; looking at myself in the mirror to see how cool I looked. I practiced holding it different ways and breathing smoke out my nose and making smoke rings. It definitely was the thing to do with some groups of people, and it paralleled drinking. When I drank, I smoked. My sisters and I used to get away from the house and the parents to go drink and smoke. They would never have allowed us to do it at home.

When I was sixteen, I got my driver's license. My parents got us a car so that I could chauffeur my sisters around. That car became the place where we smoked. We used to call it the ashtray because it smelled so horrible. The smoke would come pouring out when you opened the door. My parents knew we were smoking but they ignored it. I know they didn't want us to smoke but they probably couldn't figure out how they would be able to enforce a rule against it. My dad, every once in a while, threatened to take us down to the basement and show us slides of discolored lungs and lung cancer slides. But that didn't stop us. We only laughed at him. I knew that people died of cancer.

When I went away to college, I felt really emancipated and I could buy my own cigarettes. Previously, even though I had a car, I was only sixteen and you had to be eighteen to buy cigarettes. So we would go to certain service stations where they sold cigarettes from the service island because they wouldn't make you show an I.D. We would buy Tareytons. After I went away to school, I switched to menthol cigarettes, Benson and Hedges 100s. I'd charge them at the school store on my student I.D. I used to get a carton of cigarettes at a time, and I always protected my supply by having a carton at all times so I would not run out of cigarettes. I rarely bought cigarettes out of a machine because they were not the kinds that I liked.

I figured I would smoke through college and then I would quit. I don't know where I picked up that idea. I don't know why I thought it would be cool to smoke in college and then stop. Maybe it had to do with my parents having quit. I know my mom had smoked in college because we have some pictures of her smoking. I went to the same college that she had gone to so it may have been that I thought smoking is something that you just do while you're in college. I didn't have much conception of what life was going to be like after college, but I did think, I'll smoke through college and then I'll quit. I didn't worry too much about how I was going to quit, but there's no question I was real addicted to smoking. I was smoking two to two-and-a-half packs a day in college.

And the fewer my classes the more I smoked. I wrote my thesis by writing and smoking and typing through the entire day until one night I went to bed and I literally could not get my breath. I could taste ashes in my lungs. It felt like my lungs had turned to ashes. I knew that was real bad but here I was, in the middle of this thesis and the cigarettes just seemed like a part of it. I needed them. Colds, sore throats, whatever, didn't convince me to stop. Sometimes I'd cut back but I didn't stop.

Interestingly enough, most of my close friends were nonsmokers. I would not have tolerated the behavior from my friends that they tolerated from me. They didn't smoke but I would keep an ashtray in each of their rooms and I'd come in and smoke. I remember us going some place on the train and we had to sit in the smoking car. I was so insensitive. I wouldn't tolerate that now from people. I ask people not to smoke in my house and in my car.

But back then I wouldn't stop smoking even for a two-hour train ride. I remember smoking and drinking coffee, which I'd developed a liking for in college. My friends and I would sit around and drink coffee and smoke after meals and talk and talk and drink and smoke.

I loved smoking. It was doing for me what I wanted it to do, whatever that was, those early years in college. It didn't bother me that I was addicted, but I did expect to be able to quit at some point. I very much enjoyed my life. College was everything I dreamed it should be. I was smoking, drinking liquor and coffee, sitting around and talking with friends. And, of course, I felt invulnerable.

But I started thinking about quitting smoking

in my senior year, right after my real bad experience while writing my thesis. I was having trouble catching my breath and I knew that my lungs were in real bad shape. I had noticed that I couldn't run anywhere. I was having a hard time getting my breath after walking up a flight of stairs. Towards the end of my senior year, I decided to quit and so I got rid of my cigarettes. That lasted about a day. Then I decided I would have a cigarette now and then. My sisters were always occasional smokers. They smoked maybe three cigarettes a day. I thought I could probably do that. I went to a couple of parties and I decided that even though I was quitting smoking, I could have a couple. I remember borrowing a couple from somebody and within two or three days, I was back up to two-and-a-half packs a day. Having an occasional cigarette didn't work. It was a miserable failure. I didn't try to quit again for probably another year.

I'm glad, in a sense, that it happened that way, because I needed to understand that for some reason I was either going to do two packs a day or I wasn't going to be able to have any. I certainly was not going to be able to just smoke at parties or just have a few a day. That wasn't the type of smoker I was. That's when I got my first clue I was truly addicted. Before then I enjoyed smoking and I never thought of myself as addicted. I thought I was real sophisticated and people who didn't smoke were square.

My friends and I would sit around and have philosophical discussions and talk about ending the war in Vietnam and we'd go to demonstrations. We were very deeply and philosophically committed to things but, interestingly enough, not to our own bodies. We did not have respect for our own bodies and didn't know what we were doing to them by smoking or using LSD or other chemical substances. We were rebellious so anything that society was doing we were against. Besides, I didn't see myself going without cigarettes because I had always bitten my nails. I did that even when I smoked so I thought it would be terrible if I didn't smoke. What would I do with my hands? What would I do with my mouth? I always wanted to be doing something. I liked playing with the cigarettes. I liked taking them out and messing with them and lighting them. I always had my lighter with me and I did a lot of character playing that I enjoyed.

When I reached the point of really wanting to quit, something that helped me was yoga. I realized that it was difficult doing the yoga and doing the breathing exercises as long as I smoked. I couldn't take a breath down to the bottom of my lungs. Doing yoga cleansed me and I felt like my breathing was getting better, but then I'd light up a cigarette and I knew how contradictory that was. I finally got to the point when I said it's one or the other. I was either going to drop the yoga or the smoking. During college I hadn't been into fitness of any kind. I had the required gym and I took as little of that as I could. I took bowling once to fulfill the requirements but bowling didn't interfere with smoking.

My first attempt to quit smoking wasn't successful, and I continued to smoke for about a year after I graduated from school. I was more and more nervous about it because I was reading about how bad it was. There were many magazine articles, and I started to pay attention to them and was aware that something was happening in my lungs. I started to think a little bit more about my grandpa and worry about that. One article in particular really scared me because it talked about menthol cigarettes and how bad they were for you. The menthol sterilize cilia in your throat and the cilia, once they become paralyzed and die, are not replaced. Their job is to act as a filter in your throat. The idea that I was killing something that wasn't going to be replaced really frightened me. I was doing something to my body that was not going to grow back.

I always had the thought that when I quit I'd take control and be back to where I was before ever smoking. Now I knew different. When I thought of the thousands of menthol cigarettes that I had smoked I really got scared. Every time I lit a cigarette, I was aware that I was doing something really harmful to myself physically. I was torn. I was getting to the point where I wanted to quit more than I wanted to continue. But I had to get to the end of that process.

There was a period where I didn't like the idea of smoking. I was talking about quitting, I was thinking about quitting, and yet I wasn't completely committed to it. Finally, I think the yoga was teaching me to feel better about my body. I believed it was good to take care of it and be respectful of it. I don't remember exactly when I decided to quit, but I got to the point where everything was right. I was ready to quit and I threw away the many packs of cigarettes I had.

I was surprised that I wasn't more physically addicted. I thought I would have some real physical side effects because I'd heard about people being really crabby and having a hard time. And I didn't. It wasn't that bad. I didn't crave nicotine. I was surprised that it wasn't harder. I missed it a lot after mealtimes when I would normally sit around, have coffee, and light a cigarette. I felt a real pang that I couldn't do that anymore. But I continued the yoga and I felt good about that. Pretty soon I started to notice positive things.

I had a little more breathing capacity when walking or running. I realized my clothes didn't smell anymore. I hadn't realized how bad people smelled who smoked. However, it was years before I got around to having a nonsmoking house and a nonsmoking car and asking people not to smoke around me. One of the positive things that happened right away after quitting was the release from fear. I had really felt scared, especially about what menthol did to my system. I had been feeling uneasy every time I lit up and I knew I was doing irreparable damage. The relief was there that at least the little cilia I've got left are okay. Whatever are in there, only God knows how many are left, they're okay. I knew my lungs would turn pink again and I would think about that. It felt good knowing my lungs were getting better and better.

Quitting smoking was lonely. I didn't have any support when I quit. I did it myself. Nobody was particularly interested. At the time, I didn't have a lot of ties with people. I was just ending a job and I took a temporary job. I was planning to go to graduate school in England. My husband and I were breaking up, getting back together, breaking up, and getting back together again. I wasn't close to many people. In fact, I had no real close friends. It was a real unsettled time for me. I struggled, quitting all alone. I continued doing yoga but I didn't begin any other exercise. I felt better about my body almost immediately. I gained a little weight, probably because I ate more sweets, but that didn't seem to be a big deal. My dad had used candy to help him quit too.

From the very start, I was committed to not smoking again. There were lots of times, in the back of my mind, when I wanted to start but I had this conviction that I would have to get all my powers together to quit again. Quitting had been hard enough, so I didn't want to do that. That realization kept me from starting smoking again.

I haven't had a cigarette since 1973 or '74. I can't remember, for sure, but it was after I graduated. There was the temptation to smoke again when I went through law school. School and smoking went together. It seemed like I should be able to have a cigarette. But I knew if I lit up, I'd start smoking again. And, of course, the further on I get into my recovery from alcoholism, the more I do have supportive people and people who are nonsmokers around me who would challenge me about smoking again.

I know few people who smoke anymore. In fact, when I'm around smokers I ask them not to smoke around me. It seems that everybody I've talked to has tried to quit; the reason they're still smoking is they haven't quite found a way to quit yet.

The benefits to not smoking are great. My health is so much better, and I know that whatever else happens to me, I'm not poisoning myself. Another thing that has become increasingly important is I've gotten rid of some of the other medicators too. Smoking wasn't the only medicator.

Smoking is an incredible distraction. It keeps people away. I've asked people who smoke not to, not because the smoke was coming into my face but because their hands were always in front of their face, in the midst of a cloud of smoke. Smoking makes connecting difficult. The lack of intimacy bothers me. I've started thinking about that and thinking about what I was trying to say to people when I was giving off clouds of smoke. I know now that I was clearly hiding and wanting distance from other people.

My sister is getting a divorce, and one of the reasons is because my brother-in-law is overweight and a compulsive smoker who refuses to quit and she's afraid that he will die. She has decided she wants to be with someone who wants to live. And that's something that's important to me too. People who smoke are like people not wearing seat belts. It's passive suicide.

A tool that others might use to stop smoking is yoga. It was so cleansing. It was good to get a little bit in touch with my body. It's neat because it's not just mindless exercise which is what really attracted me to it. I had to think about what I was doing. In yoga you're a funnel of affirmation. You send affirmations, good messages, to different parts of your body, and the body responds. It's not just a passive thing.

Every once in a while I wonder if I stopped in time. Am I going to get lung cancer? My grandfather had stopped smoking when the doctors told him to and he still got emphysema. It's not reversible. I'm glad I love myself enough to have stopped. I like being a nonsmoker. I don't think there's anybody left in the whole United States of America who doesn't know that if you smoke, you're killing parts of your body. It really is an out and out statement that "I don't care about myself." I'm glad I'm not saying that anymore.

MIKE

Age 39. Professional salesman, cur-
rently selling glass products; married,
father of two; loves racquetball and
going to health clubs; is an avid
reader and political buff.

I smoked for the first time when I was nine
years old. I was on the way home from the movie
Bambi with my good friend, Greg. I was an only
child and Greg had an older brother whom we
idolized. He was about seven years older and, of
course, he smoked. Greg looked at me and said,
"Mike, do you smoke?" I said, "No," and he said,
"Want to try?" I said, "Sure." I was a straight
Catholic kid and all that stuff, but there was that
part of me that needed to rebel so we picked up
butts off the street and we started smoking although we didn't inhale until we were fifteen or
sixteen. I smoked for five years, puffing without
inhaling on cigarettes. Greg would steal them
from his dad, or we would pick the butts up off
the street or we used to buy them from an older
kid. We'd go and sit in the bushes and smoke.

I got into football and wrestling in high school
and as long as I was doing a sport, I wouldn't
smoke. But then when I wasn't doing a sport, like
when wrestling season ended, I started smoking
again. Camel straights was what I smoked because they were macho. I thought that if I'm going to smoke, I'll smoke Camel straights. I won't
smoke sissy stuff.

Funny, though, that I didn't miss them at all

when I quit. I can remember every year on June 1 I would go down to Lake Calhoun and symbolically throw my cigarettes out the window and I wouldn't think about smoking again until after wrestling.

During this entire time, my parents never had an inkling that I smoked. My mother and my father were divorced when I was two, and Mom and I went to live with my aunt and uncle. My mother never smoked that I remember. My aunt didn't smoke either. My uncle smoked for a period of five years between ages 50 and 55 and he quit. My father has never had a cigarette in his life. My home life certainly didn't influence me to smoke.

I was always trying to walk the line between being this great athlete and doing like everybody else. I never thought smoking was that great but then there was a whole side of me that involved liquor, along with cigarettes. When I got to college all hell broke loose. I began smoking, drinking, and partying all the time. By the time I entered the service, I was smoking about four packs a day. I was a paratrooper and I was running. I could run forever in the service, and I wasn't having any harmful consequences. In fact, when I got back home, I applied for a job and had to take a physical that included the Harvard Step Test. I had a relaxed heart rate of 38. I was in incredible shape, even doing four packs of cigarettes a day.

I got a job where I could smoke at my desk so I had a place where I could smoke constantly.

However, my next job was real estate and one of the things they told me in training was not to smoke with my customers, and I thought that was a good idea because I knew some people were allergic to smoke and found it offensive. So I never smoked with customers. That was my first step in breaking away. Sometimes I'd go for a day and I wouldn't think about smoking because I knew that once I dropped potential buyers off, then I could have a cigarette.

My wife quit smoking in 1977. She quit cold turkey and we both tried at the same time but it was terrible for me. I just couldn't do it. It was so difficult and the big thing I remember thinking was that when I'm not smoking, I'm not in control of my life. If I can smoke, that means I'm in control. That means I'm making the decisions. To not smoke is like Sister Mary Elizabeth telling me to do this or to do that. As backwards as it sounds, not smoking to me means that I'm not in control at all.

Before quitting recently, I controlled always where and when I'd smoke. I gave up smoking during the day, and my children never saw me with a cigarette in my hand. For about seven years I never smoked during the day. Once Shannon was born, I never smoked until 8:30 at night after she was in bed. Now that I've quit, it feels like my choice has been taken away and now I'm no longer in control of my life.

The first time I quit, a few years back, I switched to cigars for a while. Pretty soon I was inhaling them so finally I said if I'm inhaling these I might as well go back to cigarettes, so I did. However, I still never smoked with customers. I always waited until I got home.

For years, I associated relaxing with having a cigarette. When I can sit in my favorite chair and light up a cigarette then I know it's *my* time. The kids are in bed; the dishes are washed; the clothes are done. Since I've quit smoking now, even though I was down to only five or six cigarettes a night, except on weekends when I'd maybe go through a pack, I don't know what to do with myself. I don't feel like I can relax and I've been having trouble sleeping. My wife went through a nonsleeping period for quite a while too when she quit a few years ago.

I also always associated a bowel movement with smoking. I had a deathly fear that I would be constipated when I quit smoking. It didn't work out that way but I really thought it might. I had gotten into a particular routine and I expected changing the routine would cause problems.

A lot of people wondered why I even wanted to quit since I smoked so little, but a friend I play racquetball with got me to thinking about it. We go back to when we were three years old, and he quit smoking ten years ago. One day we were talking about his upcoming 39th birthday. All of a sudden we were talking about aging and it was like I was on a roller coaster and I hit a brick wall. "I'm going to be 40 years old." I started thinking about it and I realized I wanted to be around to see my kids grow up. Besides, I figured, since I was down to half-a-dozen cigarettes a day, only smoking evenings, I could easily quit.

I had another friend who was a three-pack-a-day Old Gold smoker. He and I go back 30 years. One day, four years ago, he decided to quit. He had talked to somebody about acupuncture. He tried it and it worked for him. That was it. He has not had a cigarette since, and I figured, Hey, I'm going to try that, and so I did.

The acupuncturist was from the Philippines. He was rather cherub-like. He gave me a physical and talked to me. He explained acupuncture and told me how he got into it. He said that he thought it was a bunch of bull at first but he said that when you're an internist you treat ailments and a lot of times you can't do anything for them and medications often cause side effects. He was always trying to figure out what to do to alleviate some of the side effects from some of the drugs, so he started studying hypnosis. Over a period of years, he got more and more into it and found that with some people it helped. He said if you can find anything that helps in any little way, when the medicine and the schooling fail, you latch onto it. And then a doctor friend of his went to a seminar on acupuncture and two years later was having success using acupuncture along with medical treatment. Finally he investigated it too and has had good results.

So I took his treatment and it's worked for me. I haven't smoked since. I've changed other habits too. I started going to a health club and I'm still playing racquetball. The only problem is that

I'm still so orally fixated that I force-feed about 2000 to 4000 calories between 8:30 and 10:30 at night. I'll eat a bag of Fritos or a bag of Cheetos or a bag of peanuts. Because I'm working out, I've only gained about ten pounds but if I can cut out the extra intake of calories, I'll lose the twenty pounds that I want to lose.

I still miss cigarettes, though. I love to read and normally, after the kids went to bed, I'd sit down to smoke and read a book. I've been reading my present book for about two months! I just can't get through a book. I can't concentrate. I can watch television because that doesn't do anything to affect my urge, but I cannot sit down and read even the paper. I have a hard time because I associate that activity with relaxation and I don't have cigarettes to relax with now. However, I'm determined to stay a nonsmoker.

Nobody in my family has ever had cancer so fear of that didn't haunt me, but there's a history of being short, heavy, and prone to heart attacks. My Uncle Kelly and my Uncle Eddie had heart attacks. When you have that history in your family and are prone to being overweight, you think about consequences. My grandfather is 97. Until about two years ago, he was working full days, five or six days a week. I don't know if I'll live that long but I sure would like to see my kids get through college. And if not smoking will help, then I'm committed to it.

There are some real pluses to not smoking. It isn't all hard. One of the pluses is I can play good racquetball. All of a sudden I feel I can play forever again. There's a major difference in my stamina. I know there are other rewards but I'm still trying to find them. Right now, I still feel out of control because I'm not smoking. I'm sure it's just a matter of working on that and turning it around to feel I'm in control because I'm not smoking! I just haven't made that leap yet.

The big thing I've learned about quitting is that it's not easily done alone. It helps to take all the things that can be learned in support groups or all the things that can be learned in treatment programs and apply them because nicotine is a chemical dependency just like any other chemical dependency. On the surface behaviors don't seem to manifest themselves as negatively as with other chemicals. However, you're still doing things to your body that are terrible and it's an addiction just as strong as any addiction. But I believe it can be licked, just like any other addiction, if you get help whether from acupuncture or some support group. Quitting cold turkey means changing your whole attitude and it'll never happen overnight. It's difficult. It's a difficult thing to do but if you really want to do it you can. There are benefits to quitting but you sometimes need to talk to other people to remind yourself what those benefits are. The main one for me is I can now expect to see my kids grow up.

RUTH

Age 73. Mother of seven daughters and one son; grandmother of four girls and four boys; avid reader and tennis player; commitment to volunteerism through church and community organizations.

I think I was forced into smoking by circumstances. I really didn't like smoking when I first started in 1930. I started working at a bank when I was about eighteen, right out of high school, and I was working with a bunch of young women like myself. We had a rest room that was set aside for us and everybody in that rest room was always smoking. It was the cool thing to do at that time. I tried unsuccessfully to smoke a few times and didn't like it. I would quit trying for awhile and then I would think, well, I don't really belong if I don't smoke. So I would go and get a pack of cigarettes. It took me a long time to learn how to smoke them.

Finally, by about 1932 or '33, I got pretty good at it. My sister, Bea, and I were really good friends in that period. We used to run around a lot together. We'd vacation together and she smoked. I got pretty good at it with practice.

When I got married, I was sick a lot so I just didn't smoke at all and quitting was easy. There was no stress about quitting. I don't think that I had developed a really bad habit during that period at all.

By the time I started having babies, though,

44

I'd smoke an occasional cigarette. I don't think I even inhaled. I'd just puff on them in the evening, but I never smoked during the day when I was at home. I smoked sporadically. We went out for the evening and everybody was sitting around drinking, then I would have a cigarette with my drink. It wasn't until the kids were pretty well grown up that I started buying cigarettes for myself.

I think the kids leaving home led to more active smoking. I had less and less to do. And my husband was much busier in that period. He was in the real estate business, and he wasn't home a lot. He was drinking and I was getting more and more isolated. I didn't have very many friends. I was alone a lot and I filled the hours with reading. Smoking and reading just seemed to go together.

Cigarettes were my companion, my solace. But still I wasn't a heavy smoker. I never was a heavy smoker, because I never really liked to smoke that much. I would get cigarette hangovers if I smoked more than two or three cigarettes in a row in the evening. If I smoked even half a package of cigarettes total, I'd have a terrible hangover from it. And cigarettes always sapped my energy. Instead of getting up and doing something, I'd think, well, I'll go have another cigarette. Maybe that'll make me feel better. I never knew smoking was dragging me down. During that time I had an ulcer and the doctor told me not to smoke. It is terribly hard on the ulcer. I'd go for long periods and wouldn't smoke because my ulcer was so bad.

In spite of how little it seemed, I was still smoking and had a serious nicotine habit. When we moved out of the city, I started smoking heavier. I even started buying cigarettes and smoking on my own. Smoking became a real habit. It became part of my daily life. By this time I even bought them by the carton. I smoked a pack a day which was much more than at any previous time.

I tried to quit a couple times after my habit had become full-blown. I'd quit for maybe two weeks and then I'd start again. I'd decide that smoking wasn't hurting me that much. Or sometimes I'd think the opposite. I'd decide that smoking is really harmful, and I'd just quit. I was seesawing back and forth all the time. Then one day I finally decided I wanted to quit. I *really* wanted to quit. So I did. I didn't smoke for two years and then, because of my husband's chemical dependency, I entered a family treatment program where, unfortunately, everybody smoked. My nicotine habit came back full force. I was spending more time thinking about cigarettes than I was about treatment, so I decided to start smoking again. I smoked from May until October and then I quit again. I haven't smoked now for two years.

The first time I quit smoking I ate lots of sweets that resulted in a gain of ten pounds. I quit cold turkey and it didn't seem to be that big a deal. It didn't seem a very hard thing for me to do. It must have been, though, because when I started again during treatment I had a psychological need to smoke.

This last time I quit I hadn't really planned it. I just ran out of cigarettes and I didn't buy anymore. My husband no longer smokes and it's easier not to smoke if nobody around you smokes. I did experience loss of concentration. For three or four days I couldn't settle down to anything. I would begin a project or begin reading or doing something with my hands but I couldn't stay at it for very long. I needed to get up and walk around and look out the window to get my mind off of what I was doing so that I could get a fresh start.

I missed my morning coffee, cigarettes, and the paper. That's a routine that I had enjoyed. So, when I quit smoking, I quit drinking coffee too. And I delayed breakfast. I would do something else right away when I woke up. Coffee, cigarettes, and the newspaper all went together. They were a habit and when you change your habits, you change that compulsion.

This last time I quit it was easier. I guess it was because I wanted to quit. I didn't have that leftover feeling that I ought to quit. I really wanted to quit. And that makes quite a difference.

DOUG

Age 37. A high school counselor and teacher; twice married, adoptive father of a ten-year-old boy; loves coaching Little League and a chess team; jogs, collects antique toys, and loves practical jokes.

I started sneaking around to smoke in junior high. My dad was a smoker at that time so frequently a pack of cigarettes would be laying around and I would take a couple. I knew he wouldn't miss them. And then a friend and I would go off to smoke. Sometimes we went to his basement when nobody else was around. We also hid out under a bridge where no one could catch us. We tended to seek out-of-the-way places. We feared that if somebody saw us they'd report it to our parents.

I continued smoking throughout junior high but those of us who smoked then were in a minority. Smoking was a real curious thing to do. I wasn't looked down on by my peers for trying cigarettes. It was a fun thing to try. We even tried smoking cigars. It was no big deal. However, when I got into high school, I started hanging around with a healthy group of kids and I outgrew the smoking stage for a time. In fact, I didn't smoke again until college. I didn't have a desire to smoke during my early years in college even though I hung around with both smokers and nonsmokers while living in the dorm.

And then, when I was either a junior or a

senior, I began smoking again. My roommate was a pretty heavy smoker and it seemed like I just stumbled into smoking again. It wasn't planned. Somebody offered me a cigarette in a bar and I tried it. It was relaxing and I enjoyed it, particularly when I drank. Smoking seemed to accompany the whole setting, the whole mood. I'd get a little buzz when I smoked and I really enjoyed that part too, particularly the first couple of years.

In time I began to realize it was controlling me. It more or less took over my life. By my mid-twenties I really couldn't live without a cigarette in the morning as well as throughout the day. At the time, I taught 30 miles from my home. My daily routine was to get up in the morning and have a cigarette first thing. Then I'd shave, shower, and eat a quick breakfast. During the 30 mile drive I'd enjoy a couple of cigarettes. And then at school, I'd have a cup of coffee and a cigarette before classes started. I'd smoke throughout the day, at break time, and at lunch. I was smoking a pack a day, except when drinking or socializing. Then I'd smoke more.

Before long I was smoking out of need rather than enjoyment. The enjoyment kind of left. I could really feel the aftereffects in my lungs upon rising in the morning if I had smoked too much the night before. At the time, I was in pretty good physical shape, or so I thought, but I remember trying racquetball one time. I was so winded I could hardly catch my breath early on in the game. I was playing with a good friend who said my smoking was my problem. I had played tennis pretty regularly all along, but tennis allows you to catch your wind after a hard volley. Smoking and tennis weren't that bad of a match. Up to this day, I really don't care for racquetball because of that memory. I just couldn't catch my breath.

Because of the shortness of breath and sore throat and lungs, I did quit smoking once for several months. I prepared for quitting by using a filter on my cigarettes which was designed to wean me away from the nicotine. I went through the weaning process for about four weeks. I got down to the last filter and the accompanying directions said I should be able to stop and I did. It was a relatively easy way to stop. I was off cigarettes for seven months. I put on some weight and I didn't like that. I was out of shape but this was in the late seventies, before the big push to get in shape had started. I was living in a town of about 10,000. There wasn't a YMCA or anything to get into. I even had to drive 50 miles to play tennis so I didn't do that more than once a week, and I really didn't get into shape.

I didn't remain a nonsmoker for long. Stress drove me back to smoking; a lot of stress in my personal life. Smoking just seemed to be a good crutch to fall back on. I remember my ex-wife was disappointed that I was smoking again. I was putting in long hours at work and I had a part-time job besides. I needed something to get me through this tough period in my life and cigarettes seemed like a good idea. That first cigarette, after not having smoked for several months, really shot right through my body. I got real light-headed and liked it.

For awhile I felt really good about smoking. It was a good companion. And then after only a month or two, I knew I was being controlled by it once again. I was no longer in charge of smoking. Soon I was back to smoking a pack a day and I did so until about '82.

In the back of my mind, I knew I would quit again. My dad had quit when he was about 40 or so. It was always in the back of my mind that I was going to quit too. Having a role model like my dad, coupled with all that I had read and heard about smoking, convinced me that it was a foolish thing to keep smoking. In '82 I stopped cold turkey. I had just remarried that year. My wife didn't even know that I had stopped smoking until two weeks after I'd stopped. I was very low-keyed about it because of my fear that maybe I couldn't do it. I didn't really want to tell anybody in case I failed.

My process for stopping began with a decision to stop. I played with the idea a little bit. I knew there would be a day when I'd say, "This is it." That day came in May. It was towards the end of school. I was sitting in the teachers' lounge; I had stopped smoking for a couple days and all of a sudden one of the teachers realized I wasn't smoking. He was an ex-smoker and he gave me a little bit of reinforcement. I needed that.

I really craved cigarettes during the early period. I chewed a lot of gum. In fact, *I had* to have gum and I chewed it for hours and hours. A couple months after quitting smoking, I started an exercise program and I got hooked but I bounced around between activities a little bit at first. I started swimming but the YMCA's hours didn't work well for me. So I tried running around the indoor track for a couple laps. I remember how it felt when I got to a mile, which was 28 laps around the track. That was a goal I was proud of. I kept increasing the laps and added a little exercise on the weights. Finally I got to a mile-and-a-half and then two miles. I kept increasing it and got into a structured exercise routine. I'm still committed to my exercise routine, and I'm disappointed if I don't exercise at least three times a week. Usually I work out four or maybe even five times a week. My routine includes 150 sit-ups, 50 push-ups, and a three-mile run. It's really important for me to hold on to that routine and it keeps my weight down. I left one bad habit and I picked up a good one.

I do get urges every once in awhile to smoke again. It's real unpredictable. Generally, it's when I'm around somebody who is smoking. I might be having a couple of beers with friends and it seems like smoking would be fun. If it didn't so quickly control me, I would still enjoy smoking. I was laughing with a friend a couple days ago and saying that when I get to be 70 years old, maybe I'll start smoking again. Maybe that will be my goal. If I get to be 70, I'll allow myself to smoke again. But when the urge surfaces now, I recognize it and let it pass. It stays with me a minute or maybe ten minutes, or it might even last an evening, but I just wait until it passes. Most of my friends now are nonsmokers; but some of the kids I teach are real heavy smokers, although they don't smoke in the school. They smoke outside of the building so I don't have to deal with their smoke.

There are many benefits to not smoking even though I still have an occasional urge. For one, I like knowing that smoking is no longer affecting my health. And I've begun to notice how smoke takes over a room. The smoke is everywhere and quickly it's in my clothes. I realize now I always smelled like smoke. I really enjoy not smoking because of our son. I feel good about being a healthy role model. And I like the exercise. I wouldn't have the energy to exercise as much if I were still smoking. Finally, I get a kick out of watching the cost of cigarettes going up, knowing that I'm no longer wasting my money. I quit when cigarettes were approaching a dollar a pack in the vending machines. Now I see that they're a dollar fifty or more in some machines. With the money I'm saving, I treat myself to little gifts that I wouldn't have bought before. That feels great. And I feel great!

PHIL

Age 36. An attorney by education; a drug counselor in a major treatment center by choice; married, father of a one-year-old daughter; an avid hiker, jogger, and fitness enthusiast; loves folk music and sports.

I didn't smoke much as a kid mainly because I always felt like I was supposed to be a good kid. I would occasionally sneak a few cigarettes from my dad's pack but I always felt terribly guilty about it even though I knew he wouldn't know. He was a chain-smoker. When I was thirteen or fourteen, one of the neighbor kids used to steal whole packs of cigarettes from his dad and we would go up in our tree house and smoke.

Even though I smoked once in a while, I really didn't care for smoking. One time I smoked four or five cigarettes in a row and got terribly green around the gills. I felt pretty awful and that discouraged me from smoking much more for a time. In fact, in high school I didn't smoke at all. I decided smoking was something punks did. But again, I was always trying to do the right thing and I was afraid of getting caught. Besides, my friends were all nonsmokers. I did not hang around with the wild guys in school.

When I really started smoking was my very first day at junior college. That day, our classes lasted about five minutes each. The teachers would introduce themselves and give us some reading assignments and dismiss us. We'd all file into the student commons. That was my first experience in that kind of an unstructured situation. My high school had been very traditional. It was nerve-racking that very first day meeting new people. It seemed everyone was smoking in the student commons, so I started smoking too that day and smoked the whole day long.

It felt pretty cool to smoke. I felt grown up. Here I was in college, hanging around and smoking in the student commons. It felt great. It helped compensate for some of my feelings of inadequacy. It helped me forget how nervous and anxious I was, and I immediately began smoking a fairly substantial number of cigarettes, from half to a little over a pack a day. That first summer I decreased my smoking a little bit. I guess the habit wasn't deeply engrained; however, as soon as school started, I was right back into it. I think being away from the restrictions of home made it easier to smoke. My mother was a nonsmoker and she didn't like it when I smoked. But I had quickly realized the joy of smoking because it helped me feel cool and not so anxious.

I smoked throughout college. I smoked until I was about 30 and, on the average, I smoked a pack-and-a-quarter a day. On occasion I smoked as much as two packs a day but I felt that was too heavy so I eased back. Actually, I probably always smoked between a pack-and-a-half and two packs, but I like to think it was less. I still have some denial about how much I smoked.

The main problem for me with smoking was the money. I had very little money while going to school and it was a substantial investment to keep myself in cigarettes every day. I wasn't aware or concerned about health consequences at that time and I wasn't very athletic. I had a pretty sedentary life-style. I was overweight, I smoked, and I drank. And I enjoyed my life. For a long time, I liked being a smoker.

All the time I was drinking, I never had any serious thoughts of quitting smoking. I set some goals every once in awhile — I said that since my grandpa had quit smoking at 22, then I'd quit at 22. And then 25 popped into my head and I thought I'd quit when I was 25. But I never seriously tried to quit. Smoking was just too comforting to me.

The turning point in my life came after I got treatment for my alcoholism. When I went into treatment, I was in a state of paranoia, really frightened about quitting drinking. I was going to quit smoking, too, and all of a sudden I had all this fear that I'd really wrecked myself over the years. I was sure I had lung cancer but the closest I came to quitting at that time was switching to a low tar and nicotine brand for about a day. I went back to my other brand figuring if I'm going to smoke at least it should be a good smoke until I quit. I didn't want to fool around with low tar and nicotine cigarettes that I couldn't taste.

With sobriety, my attitudes about smoking began to shift. I got to be less defensive towards people who confronted me indirectly about my smoking. When I was drinking if someone made a comment about my smoking, I would get inwardly very angry and defensive about it. For instance, one time I ran my car into a ditch and this couple came along and picked me up. When I got into their car, I lit up a cigarette and they asked me to put it out. All I could think of was what a couple of jerks. But the longer I stayed sober, the more I realized that there were some consequences. Smoking wasn't healthy. And it was expensive. I had hardly any money and I was going to go into a training program to become a chemical dependency counselor. When I was still drinking, it had never dawned on me to try to be healthy, to try to live a healthy life-style. I had always lived a fairly unhealthy life-style. I assumed that was the way it would always be for me. But as my sobriety strengthened, I realized that I did have some choices about my life-style.

Cost and health weren't the only consequences for me. Another consequence was a spiritual one. I was consciously trying to work the A.A. Third Step. I tried to follow the will of my Higher Power throughout the day to have some kind of spiritual connection. But whenever I was smoking, I did not have that spiritual connection. When I was involved in a self-seeking, pleasure-oriented activity like smoking, I was effectively tuned out from the rest of the world.

I also realized the loss of freedom. I needed those cigarettes and yet I wanted to be a healthier person, independent of compulsions. I liked going out in the wild to hike, but I realized that I couldn't. I needed to be near a drugstore.

All of a sudden that felt real confining. At about the same time I noticed that about two-thirds of the cigarettes I smoked did not even taste good anymore. They were smoked compulsively because I needed to have something to do. In actuality, they tasted awful.

I was also becoming more sensitive towards other people. I was upsetting some people by my smoking. But I knew I couldn't quit smoking. I didn't have any idea how or why. It seemed overwhelming to simply quit smoking. But I also was aware that I could use the Twelve Step program to help me stop smoking if I became willing to stop. So I became more open and asked my Higher Power for the willingness to stop. I had never actually tried to use my Higher Power to help me stop smoking up until the day I actually stopped. I kind of knew inside that if I asked my Higher Power to help me stop, I would have to make a commitment to then stop. Up until the day that I actually stopped, I had no idea I was going to quit. I only knew I was open to the possibility. I wasn't fighting it anymore. I was not trying to hang on to my smoking.

Then one day in July, I don't know the exact day, I woke up, had two cigarettes before I got out of bed, and the thought struck me that this was really stupid. Even though I'd done this countless times in the past, I realized I couldn't even get out of bed without having a cigarette or two. I was tired of the compulsion. I asked my Higher Power to help me stop smoking until 11:00 that morning, which was three or four hours away. That was as great a task as stopping for the rest of my life. I hadn't gone that long in a waking hour without smoking for years. I stopped. I made it until 11:00 and thought, well, I survived that, so let's try for the rest of the day. Again I asked my Higher Power to help me stop. I could definitely feel withdrawal. I was speaking rapidly. I was agitated. I felt almost giddy and high. I intentionally carried a pack of cigarettes around with me that whole day because I wanted to make it clear to myself that what I was doing was a choice. I've always hated to *have* to do something. Whenever I think I have to do something, I resist. I wanted to make it clear to myself that I had the choice to start smoking anytime if I wanted to. But the pack of cigarettes stayed there all day and it dawned on me that I actually wanted to stop. I went to an A.A. meeting that night and told one other person that I'd stopped, almost in a sneaky way as if I was afraid to admit to the world that I was stopping. I was afraid that I would fall back.

I was glad that at the time I was more or less self-employed doing as much or as little work as I wanted to. I needed to concentrate on not smoking for two or three days. I was glad I didn't have any stressful situations to face. The first day was pretty bad. I was real agitated. The second and third day I felt a sharp lessening of withdrawal symptoms. In fact, I was surprised that it was coming as easily as it was. I did not focus on smoking. Whenever the urge to smoke came over me, I used a little mental trick of pretending I was between cigarettes. That helped me get through the next two or three days. After about three days, I didn't feel any craving at all.

I needed a substitute for smoking and I substituted exercise. At that point in time, I didn't know I was capable of really doing exercise. I focused on doing a lot of walking. I'd choose to walk rather than drive when it was a mile or two. Walking became a substitute for smoking.

Now I have a compulsion with food but I didn't substitute food when I stopped smoking.

It is really good to feel free from the compulsion to smoke. I didn't appreciate how good it would feel until after the fact. I didn't know when I was smoking just how much I was missing by not being free from it. The further I get away from smoking, the more insane I think it is. I have not smoked for over six years and I see smoking as a very dangerous substance that kills people. I'm glad I'm not killing myself anymore.

In order to be successful at stopping smoking, I had to become open to the consequences of smoking, both to myself and others. It means reeducation. Most smokers plan to quit sometime. I always did. But I had to get really honest with myself and recognize that smoking is a pretty filthy habit. Smoke stinks up the world.

Secondly, I had to *stop* smoking before I could quit. All smokers plan to quit in a week or two weeks or three weeks or set a date, but, more often than not, that doesn't work. I had to make a decision to stop today and not kid myself into thinking I could cut down. Cutting down doesn't work for an addicted person. Quitting sometime in the future doesn't work either. There has to be the willingness to stop *today*.

One thing that I knew instinctively after I stopped is that I can't smoke one cigarette. It's absolutely impossible. I've never even dared to tempt myself with a cigarette. I don't even like picking them up because I still like the way they feel. I like the way they smell before they're lit up. Sometimes I like the first whiff off of a cigarette when someone else is smoking. I know these are all pretty dangerous cues for me. There's certainly a part of me that's still a smoker because I'm such a compulsive person. I definitely consider myself a recovering smoker. I like a lot of things about smoking. It was a quick fix, a quick escape for me.

The best thing about not smoking is that I'm not actively killing myself. It's really special that I care enough about myself that I don't want to kill myself. I like living now, and I'd feel pretty bad if I was smoking and putting my wife into that much jeopardy. I realize I'm a role model just as my dad was for me and I like knowing that my daughter has a positive role model. All of my siblings have stopped smoking too. We don't have any smokers in the family right now.

Something happened that surprised me recently. Even though I haven't smoked for about six years, I started thinking about smoking again. I was watching other people smoke and I thought I could probably just have a cigarette. I know that's false, and I was able to look at the fact that there was some stress going on in my life, particularly related to my job, and I think I was starting to look for a quick fix again. Smoking used to take me away from the problems that I had at a given point in time. So what I had to do was admit that I was having those feelings. It's important to be able to verbalize that I'd been feeling like smoking. It isn't something that I really want to go through ever again. Smoking kills, and I want to live.

CINDY

Age 37. A junior high school English teacher; married and the mother of two daughters; formerly a dance instructor and a drug counselor; committed to fitness and is a skillful tennis player; enjoys reading.

The first time I ever tasted a cigarette I was nine or so. My mom smoked cigarettes so I always associated smoking with women. I didn't know until I was much older that more men smoked than women. My dad smoked cigars and my mother smoked cigarettes. I thought cigars were male and cigarettes were female. My dad quit smoking when I was quite young. He just stopped. Period. He never spoke about it ever again. Even today if I were to ask him if it was hard to quit, he would say, "Well, that's just what you do."

The first time I smoked, my mom had tossed her cigarette butt into the bushes. Then she went in the house. It was still burning, so I crawled into the bushes, and smoked it, right in front of the picture window of the living room where my mom was sitting. She saw me puffing away. My sister, who is allergic to smoke now, tried it a couple times and coughed herself silly and hated it. She never did it again. But I remember liking it. When I was a little older, I went around picking up my mom's cigarette butts out of the ashtrays and smoking them way down. I couldn't figure out how my mom knew I was doing it.

I knew that my parents never wanted me to smoke and I was the kind of daughter who did what my parents said. And so as I got older, I never smoked when all of my other friends were trying it in junior high school. I was very adamant against it. There was very strong peer pressure to do it but I didn't. It was hard not to. I remember fighting it, and I never smoked in high school either. I didn't drink either. I was one of those "good" girls. Even in my early years of college, I dated a boy who didn't smoke. It just wasn't a thing we ever did. I continued to resist really tough peer pressure. By the time I was a senior in college, I broke up with this guy. I was searching for independence and I think, in my own mind, I was rebelling against my parents. I decided to smoke and I liked it. I didn't buy cigarettes for a long time. I would just borrow one from a friend and smoke at lunch or something like that. It was just kind of fun. It never entered my mind that I would become hooked. Never. Nobody was talking about the danger of smoking back then.

I teach junior high kids and they have this incredible belief in immortality. Even today, they have no concept of the dangers of smoking. They believe that they're in full control of their lives. And they believe that we're immortal; we're untouchable. That was my belief too.

Very quickly I moved to smoking a pack a day. I loved the taste of cigarettes. For eight years I smoked a pack a day. Consistently, from morning until night. The only time that I ever smoked more was when I went to parties. It's been ten years since I've smoked but if they could invent a totally healthy, nonsmelly, nonmessy cigarette that tasted good, I'd smoke it because I like the taste so much.

I decided to give up smoking because I could feel definite physical symptoms. There was a tightness in my lungs and my throat. I could feel a bubble when I breathed hard. I got scared. It was there for a while before I paid a lot of attention to it. That was 1977, and people were beginning to quit. Most of my friends either do not now or did not ever smoke. However, there was a time when almost everybody smoked. Several of them had already gone through stopping and it didn't seem like it was a big deal to them. But to me it was. It was a very big deal.

The first thing I did was cut back from high tar cigarettes to low tar. I had smoked Marlboro and then switched to Kent Golden Lights. My husband and I were going to quit together; I would never recommend that for anybody. Ever. Because then you're not quitting for yourself; you're quitting for them. I remember going down into the laundry room and sneaking a cigarette. I didn't want him to catch me. Then I went to those filters that you stick on the ends of cigarettes. That was helpful for me. It helped pull me away from the nicotine. By the time I finally did quit, I don't think the physical addiction was as strong. There was no question it was there, but I think trying to quit with my husband and realizing that wouldn't work made me see that I had to stop cold turkey. I simply could never have another cigarette again. And to this day I know that I cannot have another cigarette. Even now, after ten years, if I were to have one, I know I'd start smoking again. I couldn't focus on quitting for just one day at a time. For me it had to be forever.

Quitting was so horrible. I can still remember the pain. I started shaking. I couldn't concentrate on anything. I remember sitting in my office at school, talking to a student and I had to get up and leave. I was nervous on my job. I couldn't do my job because I was shaking so bad. I couldn't think about anything else. I remember telling a teacher who came into my office that I couldn't talk to her then because I needed a cigarette so badly. I needed so much to talk to people but there wasn't a support system. I used to try to talk to my husband about quitting because I needed his support but he wouldn't talk about it. He said he couldn't talk about it. I still believe a better way to get rid of some of those feelings is through talking to others. I really needed support because it was hard. It was really hard.

I felt very alone. People were happy for me that I was quitting, but I just didn't feel like I could talk about my feelings to them. It made me very sad to reveal my feelings. I felt so alone at the time. I had felt so out of control of my life.

My physical reaction lasted for eight or nine days, and then I started not to shake as much and I could concentrate better. But that first eight or nine days were so hard that I will never start smoking because I never want to go through that again. It was the most painful thing I've ever done. I hesitate sharing that with others because I don't want to scare them off. It does get better though.

About two or three months after I quit, I awakened in the middle of the night and couldn't get back to sleep. All my life I'd been a wonderful sleeper. Sleep has been very important to me. I like ten hours of sleep and sleeping late on the weekends. But I began having insomnia. It was horrible, and it lasted for a year and a half. I would have no trouble getting to sleep, but I would awaken in the middle of the night and be up anywhere from an hour to four hours a night. At the time I didn't associate the insomnia with not smoking.

After about a year of this, my husband and I started going to a therapist. Since I couldn't sleep, I was going berserk. Seeing a therapist opened up all sorts of issues that weren't necessarily connected to the insomnia. We discovered my insomnia wasn't really the problem. The problem was depression and low self-esteem. My sleeping problem was a barometer of how I was feeling about myself. It wasn't *the* problem; it was only a symptom.

What I came to understand was my insomnia resulted when I was desperately trying to get control of my life, and of me. It felt like I was trying to hold on. What I traced back to smoking was the realization that I blew out negative feelings through exhaling. I never had been taught how to deal with negative feelings while growing up. Negative feelings weren't something you dealt with in my family. And so as long as I smoked, I could get rid of them. But as soon as I quit smoking, I had no release for those feelings. And so they stayed inside. After two months, they had to come out. The therapy for me was learning how to get in touch with the feelings. I remember saying to people, "I don't get angry." But I did. However, anger in my family was wrong. Only an out-of-control person gets angry and the greatest thing you can be is in control. It was almost a moral judgment. People who were out of control were less moral than those people who were in control. Being in control was extremely important to me. Therapy for me dealt a lot with control. Smoking had allowed me to push all of that away. I never had to come to grips with any issues because I smoked and I got rid of my feelings, I thought. But they were obviously there building up. For me it was horrible to quit smoking not only because of the physical reaction but the pain of therapy too. But in the long run, the therapy was the most wonderful thing that's ever happened to me.

Other than the changes wrought by therapy, I didn't see any rewards from not smoking for about six months. I'm a tennis player and a dancer. I had taught dance for a long time. My endurance came back along with my lung capacity and my stamina. I didn't get winded. That gurgle in my throat started to go away. That gurgle was the most frightening thing. If I took a deep breath, there was a catch in my throat. That left after about six months. I knew I smelled better because I could smell people who were smoking and I realized that's what I had smelled like.

Probably because I'm a teacher, I think a lot about the education of people. And based on my own experience with quitting, I don't believe that the intellectual approach is the way to teach others to quit. People have to have information but you're never going to keep kids from smoking or any person from smoking by just giving them information. I always knew gunk came out of cigarettes. I knew very well that all that was inside my lungs, but that didn't keep me from smoking.

I stuck by my emotional decision because I kept remembering the pain that I'd gone through and I couldn't allow myself to go through that pain again. I still cannot concentrate as long as I used to. It's harder for me to read a book now and it's been ten years, practically. A book has to be much better to keep my interest. I used to use cigarettes for rewards. I'd be correcting English papers, and maybe after five papers, I'd have a cigarette. Now, a reward might just be getting up and going to the bathroom. I try and find some other little thing that rewards me.

The best part of not smoking is the freedom. When I was going to therapy, one of the things I found out was I didn't have a lot of control over anything in my life, but I was trying so hard to hold on to things. A friend of mine at that point gave me a button that said, "Thanks for not smoking." She said she wanted to remind me of the areas where I do have control. I remember crying when she gave that to me because it was wonderful support. And I also did learn that there are other areas where I don't need control and that's okay. Smoking felt like this monster holding me and to be free of that was wonderful. Now I don't feel trapped.

For a long time I had dreams about smoking, lots of dreams. In the dream, somehow or other, I had forgotten that I had quit smoking and I moved back to square one again. It was a feeling of real fear. I was disappointed in myself because in the dream it wasn't a conscious choice. It was something that just happened and so it wasn't my fault; my feeling was all of that for nothing! And then I'd wake up and feel tremendously weak.

I think the hardest time was when I wasn't seeing any reward at all. It's kind of like having a new baby. The first few months after the baby is born are horrible. There are few rewards, only dirty diapers and crying. Then all of a sudden they smile at six weeks old and it's just in time. You're ready to throw them out the window and they smile at you. One little tiny reward is enough to help you get going, and then you get more and more and more and you realize that it's only going to be getting better and not getting worse. It's the same with not smoking. Those little rewards were enough to sustain me.

Talking to former smokers and asking them to listen is wonderful support during the hard times. It would have felt less lonely for me if I'd been able to do that. I think a big thing for me was to try and figure out why I smoked. My husband and I smoked for very different reasons. Therefore, our quitting needed to be very different. I smoked for tension release. I didn't smoke for pleasure. Although I liked it, I sure didn't smoke for pleasure. There were about two cigarettes out of the day that were really pleasurable. Sitting down with a cup of coffee in the morning with the first cigarette, that was a pleasure. Sitting down with a drink and a cigarette was really pleasurable.

The smoking part of my life seems so long ago. I don't ever think about smoking now and I never thought I'd get to this point. For a long time, I'd think about smoking but then the feeling would pass. To ever start again would mean quitting again. And it was too painful. I'm willing to go through pain if there's a benefit, like childbirth. I'm willing to do that but with smoking there's no benefit.

VIRGINIA

Age 30. Medical office manager by profession; avid reader by choice; married, mother of a newborn son; a warm and compassionate woman who is talented as a seamstress.

I started smoking really young. I probably smoked my first cigarette when I was ten or eleven. It wasn't real clear-cut, my going from being a nonsmoker to a smoker, because there was so much smoking going on at our house. Both my mom and dad smoked and I had six older sisters. It was cool to smoke. I can remember that by the time I was in eighth grade, I was a regular smoker. I don't remember how much I smoked but I was buying cigarettes even though I only smoked with my friends at first. I started smoking with my sisters when we were supposed to be in church on Sunday morning. I smoked with my sisters, but I didn't do very much socially with them because I was too young.

My friends and I mostly smoked outside, and whenever somebody's mom wasn't home, we'd have smoking parties. I remember the house we lived in had a loft in the garage. My dad didn't park his car in the garage. It was used for storage and nobody ever went into the garage. That became my clubhouse. It was great; wonderful for smoking.

At school, my friends and I smoked in the bathroom. I can remember getting suspended for it in the ninth grade. My mom and dad were in

Mexico. I was really stupid because I didn't know the school's rules. If you were suspended you had to bring a note from your parents and you had to pay a ten dollar fine. I forged a note from my mother but I didn't pay the ten dollars. Before they would let me out of school at the end of the year, they said I had to pay a ten dollar fine. So my mom found out but she didn't openly acknowledge my smoking.

I started smoking pot around that same age. Two of my sisters, Mary and Rose, were still at home. When Mom would find pot, she would take it and flush it down the toilet and never say a word. It was real wierd. I don't think my mom ever acknowledged that I smoked, and I don't think I ever smoked in front of her until I'd graduated from high school and moved out, after which I was an "adult."

I can remember feeling so powerful when I first started. It was a way to be cool; to be doing what other girls that I admired were doing. I don't think I ever thought about quitting or thought that smoking wasn't good for me until I was seventeen or eighteen, and then I fell in love with a fellow who didn't smoke regular cigarettes; but he smoked pot constantly. It was 1973 and I was a hippy. I did not shave my legs. I was part of the "go back to the land" movement. Since that was my whole ideology, I did quit smoking cigarettes with hardly a struggle for about a year.

We hitchhiked across the country the year after my friend and I graduated from high school. He had dealt dope mostly, and I had worked. In those days you could live for a lot less on the road. We left town with about $600 and it lasted for three months. And we lived well by our standards. We never paid to sleep in a hotel. Sometimes we'd give people money for gas if they needed it. Most of the time not. Gas was still only 30 cents a gallon. We bought pot all the time and we bought concert tickets. We were Gypsies on the move, following the good music, and it was fun. One day, though, we had this big fight, and I went out and bought a pack of cigarettes.

I really had to work at smoking again. The first cigarettes did not taste good and they made me nauseated, but I smoked for five more years.

Smoking has always been an emotional reaction. It's almost like a haven, a safe harbor to go to. I feel such an emotional sense of loss whenever I quit. I always feel as if I've lost the best friend I've ever had. It isn't like that 24 hours a day, but I get rushes of this real emotional loss.

During those next five years I wanted to quit smoking many times and actually did quit drinking and using other drugs. Mark and I broke up, and my life changed a lot. I had a million incidents of quitting for two weeks, quitting for three months, quitting for twenty minutes. But I didn't have any plan to help me quit. I had quit once successfully with very little trauma so I didn't figure I needed a strong support system or a backup plan. I wanted to just be able to do it. I didn't want to chew Nicorette gum or go to Smokers

Anonymous or get hypnotized or have acupuncture. I said, "Well, I can just do it."

However, I was so emotionally dependent on cigarettes that I just couldn't cope without them. And for every time I quit, there's a different scenario of why I started again. After I had moved to California, I did quit for about six months and then started smoking the week before I got married. I had loved not smoking. It felt really good except that I gained about 30 pounds and that was so traumatizing. I had quit in May. We were planning the wedding. I had to pick out a dress and plan the wedding and I felt like this big, huge, fat pig. I dieted all summer and exercised vigorously, yet did not lose any weight. I was completely, utterly despondent so I started smoking again and I felt terrible, especially because my fiance had quit about two years before.

When I had quit earlier that spring, we were living together and he had expressed over and over how much he loved living in a house where nobody smoked. I knew he was bummed-out that I was smoking. I smelled like smoke and I tasted like smoke. I felt real guilty and I hid it from him for a couple days. Then I said, "Screw it!" I told him I was smoking, and we made some agreements about smoking in the house. I didn't smoke in the bedroom. I continued to smoke until October.

In October, I learned that I was pregnant, and I had always said that when I got pregnant I would quit smoking. Well, it wasn't that easy. Even after finding out I was pregnant, I continued to smoke for a couple of weeks. Then I said, "Okay, this is it!" But I was only able to stop for three weeks. I would buy a pack of cigarettes, feel guilty, and then stand over the toilet, rip them all up, and then flush the toilet. And then the next day I'd do something similar. I was out of control. It felt like I was truly powerless. It took me beating myself over the head with that for two months before I finally got it that I was totally powerless. Then I realized I could use the Twelve Steps to help me.

The first three Steps of the Alcoholics Anonymous program really helped. I got it that I was powerless. My life was unmanageable around cigarettes and I was acting insane. I knew from prior experience that my Higher Power, if called upon, would really come through and give me the strength I needed.

I went to my A.A. meeting one night and I talked about it. I told the truth and got lots of support. When I realized that I could not quit smoking, that I was so addicted it was out of my control and I could not quit, then I was able to stop. That was about three weeks ago and I haven't smoked since.

Unfortunately, I still think about smoking a lot. I quit because I got pregnant, and most of why I don't smoke right now is because my baby is growing inside of me. Lots of times when I want a cigarette, I'll say to myself, "I can smoke in six months, after I've quit nursing." Some days I think that I'm going to want to smoke some more and some days I know I'm totally done.

It's so socially unacceptable now. And my father, who can hardly breathe due to emphysema, is a real dash of cold water. I want to totally deny that there are health consequences. I've seen data that smoking can cause the placenta to break away from the wall of the uterus. That my smoking was life-threatening to my baby really got to me. Research indicates that mothers who smoke have smaller babies and there may be some long-term consequences for those children. They may never be as strong, physically, as children of mothers who don't smoke.

These last few weeks the urges to smoke have come but they haven't been overpowering. And what is so clear to me now again is how powerless I am. I can't just take a drag off somebody's cigarette because my life immediately goes out of control. It's scary to think that I might have to continue to go through this.

One problem is I don't ask for help when I want a cigarette. If I wanted to drink I would ask for help. Tobacco is worse for me. It feels like I get crazier around cigarettes than I do around alcohol. I guess part of it is that there are still places where I can go and smoke. There aren't any places I can go anymore and drink or do other drugs without somebody telling me to stop. But you can still smoke. There are enough people around who will tell you it's okay to smoke.

It feels great, today, to be a nonsmoker. I love it that I can breathe, that I can have a clear conscience right now. Having it clear really affects my relationship with my husband. When I smoked openly, like before I got pregnant, I noticed that if he and I were cuddled up on the couch being cute and I wanted to smoke, I would move away and smoke out the window or something. I didn't want to smoke him out. Smoking was really distancing. Then right after I smoked, I stayed away because I knew I really smelled like smoke. Smoking is very much a barrier between us.

One helpful thing I have been doing lately is a lot of deep breathing. When I'm conscious of my breath, I notice how good it feels to have clear passages and clean lungs. I know how sweet this air is when I'm not smoking. I have also used a subliminal tape. One side is a visualization meditation with relaxation along with some information about cleaning out your lungs and feeling good about not smoking and some positive reinforcements. On the other side you hear the ocean and subliminally you are reinforced not to smoke.

I'm not sure if my struggle is really over. I think it will come up strong again after this baby's out of my body. I feel like I'm a committed nonsmoker and I love it part of the time. But not always. I really do see it as a process. I watched my sister when she quit. It took her two years to really be done. To look at it as a process for me is more hopeful than to see it as something that defeats me.

For most people, it's not just black and white; for most people it's a series of stopping and starting. And hopefully stopping again.

BILL

Age 57. A divorced father of three sons who recently became a proud grandfather of a little girl; a computer expert by profession and hobby; he loves a rigorous game of racquetball.

I started smoking when I was twelve or thirteen because I saw other people, including my father, doing it. I stole them, to begin with, from my dad. At first, I snuck around to smoke, but by the time I was fifteen, I was a regular at it. I had a job in a grocery, so I got all the cigarettes I wanted. Very quickly I got to be the big man "on campus" because I could provide all the other guys with cigarettes. We all smoked but, interestingly, many of my friends never really got hooked on them like I did. I think it's just another example of the addictive personality. It felt good, so that's how I got started. I didn't make a decision to be a smoker but it quickly became a habit. When I was in the service, everybody smoked. I don't think I knew anybody that didn't smoke for years. Only the last ten or fifteen years, probably because of all the cancer scares, have friends of mine quit. In years past, everybody smoked.

The joy of smoking for me was sucking in a lung full of smoke, particularly the first one of the day. It gave me a little high but after two or three cigarettes, it was more of a habit for the rest of the day. I think very early on I decided smoking was a terrible thing to be doing and it was a nuisance, as well as being expensive. I was a two-pack-a-day guy from age fifteen on. But it had become a habit, and if one cigarette felt good, then two felt better. Also, I was a nervous person and smoking became a nervous habit. When I wanted to concentrate on something, I'd have two or three cigarettes.

Not until my later years of smoking when it became a health problem did I seriously begin to question what I was doing. In many places where I planned to smoke, I couldn't smoke. More and more often, people were objecting to it. For a time I smoked pipes instead of cigarettes. I thought pipes were healthier. Unfortunately, I was doing a lot of flying and, of course, on planes I couldn't smoke a pipe, only cigarettes. But I never consciously thought of quitting until I was convinced that smoking was a hazard to my health, and that was after I'd gotten into Alcoholics Anonymous. Like a lot of people in A.A., I decided to quit everything all at the same time. I went into a halfway house after treatment with plans to quit cigarettes and coffee. The first thing they told me was that cigarettes were available and I didn't have to pay for them. I quickly got over my plan to quit smoking.

People who started smoking back when I started never questioned whether it was good or bad for you. In fact, I'd discovered some real benefits. Smoking calmed me down. It gave me something to do. And it was preferable to drinking. Until I got convinced it was a health hazard, it was a positive factor in my life, even though the expense grew and I did get people mad at me, particularly my ex-wife because I got burns in my clothes. She always complained about the smoke too. I never believed her until I quit. Now when I go into a place where people smoke, I can smell it. I sure didn't believe that when I was smoking, though. I was surprised to realize how much I had stunk as a smoker.

In actuality, it took me a long time to quit smoking. My first plan to quit was in '69 when I went into the halfway house. I didn't quit though. I moved to Texas in '70 and, shortly thereafter, in early '71, I started going to doctors because I couldn't breathe. They never told me I had emphysema but they put me on medication to help me breathe easier. I switched to pipes for a while and then I rolled my own for a while because that's tedious and it takes longer to get a cigarette. I knew I'd smoke less by that process.

The doctors told me to quit and I knew I had to. I believed it was back in '71, but I was so addicted it took me much longer to do it than I'd figured on.

Back in Minnesota, in '72 or '73, I went to a nonsmoking clinic with a friend. We were trying to quit together and neither of us were successful, although at first I believed I would be. The smoking clinic was a behavior modification approach. We went to meetings once or twice a week and talked about our experiences. It was similar to A.A. We were to taper off from smoking by having to smoke one less cigarette every day. It seemed to work for a little while but I never had even 24 hours without a cigarette except when I had bronchitis. It didn't last. In a matter of weeks I was back up to four or five packs a day.

For a time I was on and off, always trying one thing or another to quit. I tried graduated filters, the kind where by the end you can hardly pull air through it, let alone draw smoke. I switched from regular cigarettes to filters with low tar. Towards the end, I was smoking Carltons. They were still more than enough to stir up my emphysema. Actually I was never diagnosed as having emphysema in the late '70s; I was simply on medication for breathing. I had to take a pill twice a day, and if I didn't take them, I might as well have stayed in bed because I couldn't breathe or move around. There was a rather long period when I knew I had to quit.

Although I had, in general, liked smoking, I did have some dangerous consequences, but they also resulted from my drinking. Once I passed out from being drunk while I was smoking. I had only been married a short time. I burned the mattress up and burned a hole in a fancy mattress cover. My ex-wife carried that cover around for fifteen years and used it to guilt me about my smoking or whatever she wanted to guilt me about. Aside from that, I got real good at smoking; for instance, I could light a smoke while riding a motorcycle going 60 miles per hour. I never figured out how to smoke them underwater though.

By the time I decided to quit, I looked into hypnosis. I knew about acupuncture and aversion therapy. And I decided to pick the cheapest method for quitting first. I was aware that maybe I couldn't get rid of the addiction but I was sure going to try everything that was available to do it. Hypnosis was what I tried and fortunately it worked.

The hypnotist was a medical doctor from the university. I researched it a little bit before I made my appointment. I had to wait a couple of weeks to get in, and I was determined to give myself all the odds; the day before I was to be hypnotized, I went through my apartment and collected everything that had anything to do with smoking: my matches, pipes (I must have had 70 or 80 pipes), half a dozen pipe racks, lighters, pipe dampers and pipe cleaners, tobacco, and a cigarette rolling machine. I collected a whole box full. I put everything I could find in there except one pack of cigarettes that I needed to get me through to my appointment. I gave it all to the Salvation Army. Everything. My goal was that when I got back home from the hypnosis session there would be nothing that I could smoke, literally nothing. I smoked my last cigarette walking over to the doctor's office. I threw the rest of the pack in the garbage can.

The hypnosis session was very interesting. The doctor gave a nice long explanation of what he was going to do and why, and how he felt it was going to work. He said that the main problem with people smoking is not so much the addiction; he said it's a habit. He pointed out that you make this arm motion, lifting a cigarette from an ashtray to your mouth maybe five or ten times per cigarette. If you're smoking 100 cigarettes a day, you're making that motion 400 or 500 times. He said that I had to do something about that motion. The point of his hypnosis was to remove the need for making that arm motion. He said, "I can't do anything about your nicotine addiction. You're going to have to live through that. But I can take care of the arm motion and give you a suggestion that you don't need to make that motion again." What he said made a whole lot of sense to me. He asked me as an afterthought if I was at all worried about my weight. I said I'd been trying to lose weight for a long time. He asked me how much I wanted to lose. I said ten pounds would be nice. "All right," he said, "we'll do that."

I swear I was completely aware of everything that was going on the whole time I was under his "spell." But I'm told one always thinks that. Anyhow, the bottom line is that I have never smoked since. And the first month that I quit smoking I did lose ten pounds! I gained it back but that was three or four years later. My friend was quitting at the same time and she's still mad at me because she gained the ten pounds that I lost. Hypnosis worked for me. I've sent several people to that doctor, and it's about 50/50; it works for half the people that get hypnotized, and for the other half it doesn't.

My craving was gone completely. I thought about cigarettes occasionally but I didn't have to smoke. It was similar to what happened to me with my drinking. I tried for years to quit. I went to A.A. for a year while drinking. Then I was able to quit when the right time came. I don't think either addiction would be gone if I hadn't tried all those ways to quit, but when it finally happened it was clear-cut. There were no physical symptoms, no withdrawal.

In the years since I quit smoking there have been some definite physical changes for the better. One that I never expected was I used to have headaches practically every day. I don't have those anymore. I asked the doctor about it and he said it's not uncommon for people to quit having headaches. And, of course, I can breathe. I don't have to take that medication anymore. I'm calmer, I think, than I used to be. I've had to learn to deal with the nervousness without having to use a chemical. I've begun to rely on spiritual meditation rather than medication.

The financial benefit of not smoking is great. Cigarettes now cost a buck and a quarter a pack or more; five packs would be more than six dollars. That's what I smoked some days. There's a definite benefit. I can remember being so delighted on that first day and second day of not smoking. It looked like I wasn't going to have to fight the negative consequences anymore. Quitting offered a pure benefit once I got there.

I'm a very grateful, nonbelligerent ex-smoker, and I'm very compassionate towards people that have to smoke. It hurt me so much for so long and it was so hard for me to quit that I can't help but feel sorry for anybody who's going through it.

It's so much more comfortable being a non-smoker. There are so many places where smoking is discouraged if not flatly prohibited. It's kind of nice not to have to worry about that kind of thing. I don't have to worry about whether I'm in a smoking or nonsmoking section. It's a freer, more comfortable way to live. I no longer have to check my pockets when I go out to see if I've got enough cigarettes or get up at three o'clock in the morning and go to the store. The world's becoming more and more a nonsmoking environment. There are whole companies now that prohibit smoking. The company I work for hasn't gone quite that far yet but they're going to in the not-too-distant future.

It's easier, it's really easier in the society that we live in today to be a nonsmoker.

KAYE

Age 47. A bookkeeper who is a whiz at bridge and quilting and who always takes time for friends in need of emotional support.

I grew up with smokers. Both my parents smoked so it seemed an acceptable thing for people to do, but I disliked it intensely when they smoked in the car. Sometimes I would get violently ill from it. Because of that, I made a decision, while yet a child, that I would not smoke. However, that decision was overruled when I went away to college. Their no smoking rule invited my defiance. It was grounds for dismissal if we were caught smoking. I waited until the last week of school my first year before smoking, but then I did it and I kind of liked it. It was fun and daring. I remember using all sorts of tricks to make the smoke go up, not under the door. Although it made me feel dizzy, for some reason I began to think it was sophisticated. Over the summer I worked at a resort and I experimented a lot with smoking.

At parties we'd smoke and get real high on cigarettes. I loved the dizziness. I can remember walking up the stairs and feeling giddy. I loved the feeling. I quickly became hooked and I didn't consider not smoking for probably fifteen years. I was a heavy smoker, smoking two to three packs a day depending on whether I was drinking or what I was doing at the time. And I liked every minute of smoking. For years, even when I had a cold, I loved the feeling.

My ex-husband smoked and most of the people that I dated and were friends with smoked. Nobody ever questioned smoking then.

However, over time I developed a cough and it was persistent. I couldn't get rid of it. So at about 35, I quit the first time. I signed up with a friend for a Seventh Day Adventist lecture designed to help you quit smoking. My friend didn't go to the lecture, but I went anyway. One of the things they recommended was eating oranges and prunes. I immediately ate a whole bag of oranges and a whole box of prunes. I got violently ill and could neither smoke nor get out of bed for three days. The experience took away my desire to smoke and I was off cigarettes for six months.

During those six months, I loved not smoking. My cough went away and I felt much healthier. I had a lot more energy. But one day a friend came over and she had a cigarette. I just wanted to taste it. I took one puff and that was all it took to get me started again. I was incredibly ashamed of starting again. I kept my smoking hidden from others for about a week. Then I had to let them know that I was doing it because I couldn't stop smoking. I smoked again for about a year, all that time wanting not to smoke. I just couldn't ever get to that point of thinking of not smoking again. Then I developed a cold which was so bad I could not smoke. That helped me over the hump and I quit again for about four months. Not smoking was actually easy after making it through the first three days. Once again, I felt really good. I didn't gain weight and I had a lot of energy. Most of my friends continued to smoke so I didn't have many people supporting my not smoking, but I didn't seem to need the support.

Then I went through a crisis with a friend who also had quit smoking. There had been a death and we had to arrange the funeral. That so unnerved me. I felt like I wasn't able to handle it. Because of stress, my friend started to smoke and I decided I would just smoke cigars for a time and then quit after this time passed. I was sure I could break that off. I knew if I took a cigarette I'd go right back to full-time smoking. I smoked little cigars and big ones. I smoked at work. My co-workers thought it was strange but I didn't care. I smoked wherever I was, inhaling all the time. My lungs began to really hurt, but I loved cigars. Then I began to get afraid. I'd heard that if you inhaled cigars, it was really dangerous and I was inhaling and I couldn't stop. Naturally, I started smoking cigarettes rather than endanger my health with cigars. I loved smoking from that moment on. I absolutely loved it but I felt guilty about doing it. What I began to feel the most guilty about was the damage I was doing to other people.

I remember smoking around an asthmatic. I had to talk to her from another room, talk around corners to her, knowing that I couldn't quit. Friends began telling me how much my smoking bothered them. They told me my house smelled awful from smoke, and I began to get embarrassed. I was also beginning to have some severe consequences. Another friend and I set a house on fire while smoking, and yet I didn't quit. Another time, I set my own hair on fire. The money I was spending on my habit really bothered me too. But I didn't quit again for another seven years.

When I thought I was ready to quit, I made an appointment with a hypnotist. I'd known others who had quit this way. I had to make the appointment weeks ahead. When the time came for my appointment, I cancelled it and felt really bad. I just didn't have the strength to go through with it.

Six months later, while driving to work on really icy streets, I started to hyperventilate. I got real scared and noticed that the cigarettes were making me even more afraid. That was the first time I'd ever realized that smoking made me nervous. It did not calm me down like I had always thought. I decided that I would never smoke again while driving when it was icy. That decision felt good so I decided to take it one step further and never smoke in the car.

On that same icy day, I read my horoscope and it said that whatever I started would be successful. I decided that I didn't want to go through a heavy withdrawal from smoking. I would just cut back and see if I could do that. I only smoked one cigarette every hour that day. The next day I smoked one every two hours but that's all I thought about. After about a week, I'd gotten down to two cigarettes. I was literally climbing the walls. I didn't know what to do. I had a friend who was quitting at the same time so I called her and we talked and talked. That helped a lot. I think it is really important to find somebody that has quit smoking and knows what it's like because that first week I really wanted to smoke. I felt really off-the-wall. The only place that I had never smoked before was in bed. So when I wasn't going to work or at a party with friends, I'd go home and jump in bed. That phase lasted about a week.

I was still struggling and a friend suggested I think of myself as a nonsmoker rather than as a smoker who had quit. Doing that was a real help. Another thing that helped at the time was envisioning myself in heaven going to the smoking section. It helped me to think I would eventually be able to smoke again, even though not in this life.

Unlike the previous time I'd quit, this time I did not feel physically good. I got colds and I felt deprived so I rewarded myself with sugar. Rewards are important. The first time I quit, I rewarded myself by buying jewelry with the money I saved by not smoking. This time I craved desserts and rewarded myself with them. Even after eating a big meal I never felt full that first year after quitting smoking. I was hungry all the time. Finally I had the strength to quit the desserts after awhile but not before I had gained 25 pounds. I felt heavy and unattractive and my clothes didn't fit. Physically I didn't feel any better for not smoking and emotionally I was a wreck. I almost lost my job because my emotions were so crazy that I created a scene at work and got into big trouble. I didn't understand what I was doing. I felt out of control. The consequences of not smoking were very rough for a while, but I didn't want to go back to smoking. I didn't want to be addicted to anything.

I was particularly upset about the weight I gained, but a friend assured me I would lose it eventually and I trusted that. After a year I had lost part of the weight, and after another year I lost the rest of it without dieting. I thought it was very important to go through the struggle regardless of the pain. I had been using smoking to cover my emotions. I knew if I wanted to know who I was, I had to forge ahead even though it was painful, very painful.

Today I do know myself and I like myself much better. Prior to quitting, if I was upset about something, I would smoke rather than deal with it. Now I've learned that I have to deal with the issues that surface. Maybe it means accepting some anger and trying to work it out in some constructive way or at least admitting that I'm angry. I know now I have to do something other than sit on my feelings.

I haven't smoked now for five years, but periodically, if I'm doing something that I had done as a smoker, I'll want a cigarette. A couple of years ago I went fishing and all the while we were fishing, I wanted to smoke. I had not fished since quitting smoking and the two were very related in my mind. Sometimes the urge is incredibly overwhelming. It just feels like I can't stand not smoking one minute more. But the urge lasts for no more than a minute and it goes away. Generally I don't know why the urge is occurring, but I assume something from the past triggered it. Urges come less frequently now; in fact, I don't think about smoking for months on end.

What's been best about not smoking is that I'm more in touch with myself and I love the freedom. I don't have to constantly think to see if I have enough cigarettes or where the matches are. I no longer wake up in the middle of the night and have to smoke a cigarette before I can get back to sleep. I no longer have to make sure I can stay for a whole movie without smoking. I'm beginning to feel better now, health-wise. Mentally, I feel different too. Not having to smoke gives me more time to myself. At first that was real hard for me. For instance, I couldn't just sit down and watch it snow. I had to keep moving. Now I can do that, but it's in a different way. I'm *watching* the snow; I'm not just sitting and smoking. I'm much more in touch with what's around me.

What I learned was that, to become a happy nonsmoker, it helps to think of myself as one. It's not easy at first but it is possible. Getting support from others, particularly groups, was crucial, but if I could do it all over again, I wouldn't eat sweets. It gained me nothing but some extra pounds that I had to lose.

ROBYN

Age 33. Professional dog groomer who owns her own business; enthusiastic about old cars, loves gardening, animals, boating, and physical fitness; married to a firefighter.

At fifteen I experimented with one, maybe two cigarettes in a friend's basement and didn't like smoking. But at sixteen my friends and I started running around. We had our driver's licenses so we'd go out for an evening of socializing and buy a pack of cigarettes to take along. We'd all buy cigarettes and it was fun. Early on I limited my smoking to special occasions. But within a short time, I was smoking every weekend along with drinking. That I was only a teenager didn't deter me. My mom and dad no longer smoked and they were terribly against smoking, so I didn't want them to know I had started. When I moved out of the house, at age seventeen or eighteen, I became an everyday smoker.

I became really hooked on cigarettes right away. Smoking was a big part of my life, and I loved it. Occasionally, I'd smoke a cigarette and it wouldn't taste good but not very often. Most of the time it tasted wonderful. I smoked a lot when I was nervous or sad. Cigarettes were my best friend. They were there with me all the time. They never deserted me. But I saw how they controlled me. I wasn't free to run into town to go to the store or to get gas without first finding my cigarettes and my lighter and putting them in my purse. I didn't like that but I kept puffing away.

Drinking and smoking paired up in my life. I smoked a lot when I drank. I normally smoked a pack-and-a-half of cigarettes a day if I wasn't drinking and didn't go out in the evening. But when I went out and partied, I would smoke a pack of cigarettes in two or three hours. Drinking really increased my smoking. The morning after, I would wake up and my lungs would feel awful. I think smoking a lot of cigarettes contributes to the hangover.

On a number of occasions, I wanted to quit smoking and I tried. The first time I quit was about ten years ago, at age 22. I became worried about my health. I knew that if I smoked long enough, cigarettes would kill me. Everybody, all smokers, know that cigarettes are going to kill them. But for years I was just so addicted that I didn't think about it. I'd put it out of my mind and smoke anyway. My first husband, who was many years older, smoked three or four packs of cigarettes a day. Our house was a smoke factory. He perpetually smelled like a cigarette and he had one with him constantly. I didn't want to end up like that. I was afraid if I kept smoking I would end up smoking that many cigarettes in a day, so I quit. I did not smoke for a full year.

Even though my husband kept smoking, he was very supportive of my not smoking. I needed that. When I really felt like having a cigarette, he'd say "Oh, don't. I know you really want to quit. You'll be sorry." His support helped a lot. Mom and Dad were really supportive, too, because they had quit and wanted me to quit. I worried about gaining weight and the first time I quit, I gained about ten pounds. But I still felt good about quitting.

I went back to smoking when my marriage started falling apart. I began drinking more and my inhibitions were gone. One evening I picked up a cigarette thinking I would just smoke when I drank. And that's how it started. Every time I drank I'd smoke, and for a while that was enough. However, it was not long before I got up in the morning and wanted a cup of coffee and a cigarette. I gave into the desire very soon. And in no time I was smoking more than I had smoked before I quit.

I continued to smoke another seven years but then quit for three months. I had remarried and my husband's niece moved in with us. She and I drank a lot together. She smoked too and before long I started smoking when I was drinking. Soon I was right back to heavy smoking. I hadn't given not smoking a chance.

The next time I quit, my husband and I were getting ready to go on vacation. He quit, but he didn't tell me he had quit. One day I noticed he wasn't smoking. I was really excited that he quit because I wanted to also. However, he wanted me to wait a month before I quit so he could get it under his belt. He feared we would really get on each others' nerves due to our tension over not smoking. So I waited the month, and then I quit. We went on vacation free of smoking — but I relapsed within six weeks. My drinking really triggered it. In fact my drinking triggered it every time. I'd be okay until I got a beer or a drink in my hand and then I'd want a cigarette.

Quitting this time feels different. I really want to take control of my life. Drinking was controlling me. Nicotine was controlling me. I decided that the only way I was going to be able to quit smoking was to quit drinking too. I don't know that I really thought of myself as an alcoholic initially, but I decided the only way to quit drinking and feel good about it was to go to Alcoholics Anonymous. I went to a meeting and discovered that, in fact, I was an alcoholic. I am an alcoholic. I have alcoholic drinking tendencies and if I keep drinking I will end up in very serious trouble with alcohol. So I quit drinking five weeks ago. At first, I thought maybe I should wait a little longer before I quit smoking, but I feel so good about not drinking that I feel strong enough to tackle my tobacco problem too. I quit smoking ten days ago by going to a free stop-smoking clinic at the hospital.

There were probably 25 people who went to the first meeting. There was a group leader, and it was real informal. It was similar to an A.A. meeting in that everybody introduced themselves and told a little bit about their smoking habit and why they wanted to quit and if they had tried to quit before. The leader explained the program which included setting a quit date. We talked about cigarettes being our best friend and how difficult it is to quit smoking. Many of us shared our worries about gaining weight.

97

We go to four meetings, one a week for a month, and they last about two hours. Originally, I set my quit date for a week after the first meeting. However, I had a bad cold at the time and I went home after the first meeting and coughed all night long. I thought, this is stupid. Why am I waiting a week to quit smoking? I really wanted to quit. I had made up my mind that I wanted to quit. So I decided to quit immediately. I woke up the next morning and used what I had learned in A.A. about asking my Higher Power for help. The desire to smoke was taken away. Every time I wanted a cigarette, which was quite often those first few days, I asked my Higher Power to take the desire to smoke away. And it was gone! I know it helped that I had made up my mind to quit.

I still have the cough because of a cold but it's getting better. I'm coughing up a lot of phlegm but the doctor at the smokers' meeting said that it's helping to clear the lungs faster. He advised us to breathe deeply and to do lung exercises. He said the lungs do recover in most cases. Unless you've smoked for 40 or 50 years, you'll recover almost 100 percent providing you have not contracted emphysema or some other serious disease.

Many neat things are happening to me as a nonsmoker and I think a lot of it has to do with the A.A. program. I'm getting in touch with myself and my real feelings and letting them be known. Before, I never did. I drank and smoked and just hid inside myself, from myself. I am getting in touch with why I feel the way I do about certain things and I'm talking to myself and other people about this. Before, when I wasn't drinking, I would smoke if I felt down. I'd not think about things. I'd just smoke cigarettes. But now the feelings are present.

Sometimes my feelings frighten me a little bit but I feel physically much better. I smell better. In fact, everything smells better. Food smells better and it tastes better, too, which is kind of scary because I want to satisfy that oral longing for something in my mouth. Food seems the natural substitute, but I made up my mind that I was not going to gain weight when I quit. I don't really feel hungrier than I used to except that when I felt those hunger feelings before, I covered them up with cigarettes. If I really didn't want to eat, I'd light up a cigarette and smoke and drink a Coke or something. Now I've made up my mind that if I eat something, it's going to be nonfattening, perhaps carrots or celery.

I chewed a lot of gum those first few days off of cigarettes. I don't care much for gum, however. I've used Certs. If I'm in a certain situation where I know I would have smoked in the past, I'm removing myself from that situation. For instance, after dinner instead of sitting at the supper table and smoking a cigarette with my husband, I get up and clear the table immediately and start dishes. Otherwise it's too painful for me to sit there and watch him smoke a cigarette. Instead of sitting there eating another helping while he's smoking a cigarette, I just get up. I think that eventually I won't have to do that but right now quitting is still too new and I do have to take precautions. An exceptional reward from not smoking is that I can sleep a half hour longer in the morning. I don't have to have time for coffee, cigarettes, and the paper. I don't get the paper read in the morning anymore, but I know I'd be feeling deprived if I couldn't have a cigarette while having my coffee and reading the paper, so I'm just not placing myself in that situation. I am changing my patterns. I'm taking control. The nicotine is no longer in control, and that feels good. I feel really good. I've never been in control of cigarettes before and now I am.

So many things have changed in such a short time. I was feeling really bad about my work situation. There were a lot of things that needed to be dealt with there and I was not dealing with them. I was letting my whole life slip by me, not taking control of it, passively thinking, instead, that's the way life is. I drank and I smoked and I just put up with things. I'm finding out life is what you make it. Life is exciting when I take charge and do what I want. I've always heard people say you can do whatever you want. I've always heard that. My dad always told me that I could be whatever I wanted if I put my mind to it. I never believed it, but it's true. And I'm learning now that I can do whatever I want with my life. If I can quit smoking, I can do anything. Quitting smoking and quitting drinking are just the first steps for me. I feel excited about my future, at last.

It's funny. I never expected to be saying these

things. I had watched my grandmother die of lung cancer even though she'd quit smoking probably fifteen years earlier. She discovered she had lung cancer six months after she retired. They removed a lung but it had already gone into the lymph glands and then it recurred elsewhere. She died a horrible, horrible death, a miserable death. I watched her die and I smoked the whole time. That's part of the denial of cigarettes. I was so hooked on them that I just denied that it could happen to me.

I was able to watch her die and still smoke. I can't believe I did that. Her death really did affect me and I kept thinking, I've got to quit, I've got to quit, but I put it off and put it off. Finally over a year later, I'm doing something about it.

To handle the oral fixation, I eat carrot sticks; I bring to work what you call "rabbit food." I bring broccoli, cauliflower, a dip, and maybe a banana — things that I really enjoy eating that take time to eat. I'm satisfying my hunger and I'm not putting weight on. I'm doing healthy things for myself. I'm eating food that really is good for me and the health aspect of it is real exciting. I'm doing good things for my body and my body feels better. I'm really into being healthy now when I never was before. I always thought people who jogged and did all that crap were weird. You know, now I'm exercising too! Getting healthy is exciting; it's fun, and the future excites me.

JOYCE

Age 51. Divorced mother of four; sorority house mother finishing a liberal arts degree at a major university; talented tennis player who has discovered a love for art history.

I first smoked cigarettes, while still in junior high, in what the kids in my neighborhood called the "back field." But I didn't regularly smoke until age sixteen. I was out with a boyfriend and we were on some swings on a porch. He smoked Lucky Strikes and he asked me if I wanted one. I took one and knew that cigarette was more serious than the "back field cigarettes." It made me dizzy, and I felt that between the swinging and the cigarette, I was going to get sick. But I had no thought of not doing it again. I believed smoking was something to get used to. My father and mother both smoked. However, I always felt disdainful of the way mother smoked. She didn't inhale and I always thought she looked dumb. I snuck cigarettes from my dad's pack because I didn't have much money.

Sometime during that sixteen-to eighteen-year-old period, I got hooked. I recall a car accident when I was about sixteen or seventeen and immediately after the crash, my first thought was, where are my cigarettes? I knew even then that it was a very strange thing to wonder because I'd almost been killed.

I think I was hooked on nicotine almost right away. In my family, I was forbidden to smoke in front of anyone until I was seventeen, so on my seventeenth birthday I lit up at the dining room table just like my parents. What a rite of passage that was. It really was the sign that I had become an adult.

I thought smoking was sexy and glamorous, and it was wonderful to be on a date and have the boy do like Humphrey Bogart and put two cigarettes in his mouth and light them with one match.

For years, I thought of cigarettes as my best friend. I loved smoking. I smoked first thing in the morning and the last thing at night and a whole lot in between. My children hated it. I have four children and I can remember that every time we would get in the car and I would light up, they would start coughing and fanning the air. I would get so angry at them.

For 32 years I smoked. That's a lot of cigarettes, at three packs a day, and a lot of money. During those 32 years I tried to quit a couple of times. Once, about eight or ten years before I successfully quit, I went to an American Cancer Society no-smoking clinic and made it through five days of not smoking. I had started getting a little scared because of the Surgeon General's reports. I knew cancer could happen but, in reality, I didn't think it would happen to me. But just in case, I thought I'd quit. It didn't work. Those five days were terrible. I felt like I'd lost my best friend and I didn't know how to cope with the grief of that. I had no coping skills at all. The doctor told me to take more Valium until I was over the hump.

A few years later I tried to quit another time, on my own. I created a little tool to help myself. I made a bracelet out of a piece of leather with twenty colored beads. Every time during the day that I didn't smoke a cigarette, I moved one of those beads around. I made it about the same length of time, five days. I remember coming home from work and throwing myself on my bed and saying, "What's the use? I don't even want to live if I can't smoke." I cried a whole lot and then I had a cigarette. I felt better immediately.

For a year or two before I successfully quit, I smoked the long brown cigarettes. I was working as a secretary, and every time I would type, the cigarette would go out in the ashtray and I'd have to light it again, sometimes as many as ten times. I'm not sure if relighting the stale cigarette or something else was causing it, but I started to develop a really bad cough. I got a cold and then it went in to bronchitis. Even when the cold was gone, I kept coughing. It went on for weeks and weeks. People at work could hear me coughing. It was embarrassing to me that I'd get through one of those coughing spells and then I'd light a cigarette. It seemed so abusive to myself but I was addicted. Also, by then I had been sober for a while and I had learned what it meant to be abusive to myself. It was beginning to be clear to me that there was something wrong with the way I was living my life.

The cough kept up for quite awhile, and I was really scared because it wouldn't go away. I could understand coughing while I had the cold but it worried me that it lingered and lingered and lingered. Friends began expressing concern about my cough. It was very deep and I was scared.

Where I worked, one by one the women had been giving up smoking. There were maybe six of us left, out of 23, who were still puffing away. I was beginning to get annoyed at restaurants that I was singled out as a smoker. It always seemed to take longer to get seated. I was starting to feel the difference between myself and nonsmokers, and I felt defensive and ashamed.

What helped me most when I finally quit smoking was having gone through a real difficult recovery from alcohol and other drugs and then going through an absolutely brutal divorce. I realized that although I had survived the worst pain I had ever been through in my life, I was going to kill myself with cigarettes. It didn't make any sense to me and it made me really angry. I used to say, "I didn't go through all this pain to kill myself with a cigarette now!" That's where my resolve came from. I'd already lived through a couple of little deaths. And I figured I could make it through another.

I didn't realize how effective the steps I took to quit were going to be, but I started doing some imaging of myself as a nonsmoker prior to being one in actuality. I had heard a tape about goal setting and it talked about imagery. It suggested making a scrapbook of my goals so that they would be tangible and I could look at them and start to realize them in my head. I cut out a picture of a woman smoking a brown cigarette, the same as I smoked. Then I found a picture of a big red stop sign. I pasted the stop sign on top of the woman smoking. I also cut out some other pictures of a car I wanted and a house and a man too. I began imaging the picture of the woman a lot. The image would just come to me. Apparently that helped, because the day I quit smoking, I had no plans to quit at all. I hadn't made a date yet. I was coming home at ten o'clock in the morning and I was smoking the last cigarette in my pack. It was a very cold January day and for the first time in my life, I just didn't feel like stopping for a pack of cigarettes. I knew a friend of mine was coming over in a little while and she smoked. I figured I could wait an hour until she got there, which was pretty unusual.

I finished that cigarette and I waited for my friend to come. It turned out that she didn't get there in an hour; she got there in an hour and a half, by which time I was pretty anxious. When she got there she didn't have any cigarettes either. We talked about taking a walk around the lake and decided to try the walk without a cigarette, both of us. By this time, she was getting interested in how long I had been without a cigarette. We walked around the lake and then it was probably two and a half to three hours without a cigarette and I decided to keep going. Since I'd made it three hours, I figured I could make it a little bit longer. I've never had a cigarette since.

It was awful at first. I didn't like it at all. That first night I went out to dinner and it felt like I was taking one of the greatest pleasures away from myself. I can remember sitting in that Chinese restaurant when I was all done eating and drinking some tea. I felt pretty gypped. But still, I realized that I'd gone through half a day and I hadn't come apart at the seams so I decided to keep going with it.

When things got really hard for me, friends suggested I work the A.A. Twelve Steps, but that didn't work for me. The thing that made the most sense to me was that I had gone through so much in my life to be a healthy, strong woman and I didn't want to kill myself anymore with alcohol and other drugs, bad relationships, or cigarettes. My resolve was very strong. I kept using imagery, seeing that woman in my mind. I can see her yet. I was tempted strongly two weeks after I'd quit smoking. I had a major crisis and I went out and bought a pack of cigarettes. I bought Barkley which I'd never smoked in my life. I knew someone who was trying to quit smoking and he smoked Barkleys. It made perfect sense to me. They have a lot less tar and nicotine. I didn't ever unwrap the pack. I met a friend at the movies that afternoon. She was someone I worked with and she knew that I had just quit smoking. I met her in the lobby at the movie and confessed that I'd just bought cigarettes. She put her hand out and said, "Want to give them to me?" I did. After the movie I said good-bye, went into a store and bought four candy bars and ate them all on the way to another friend's house.

I began eating a whole lot of food that had sugar in it and I put on twenty pounds in two and a half weeks. I really substituted one thing for another. But I still felt that as long as I wasn't smoking I'd worry about taking weight off later. I knew if I weakened because of gaining weight, and went back to smoking, I was caught forever. I would always have an excuse then. I never smoked and I hated gaining the weight. My body image was very important to me and the extra pounds caused a lot of pain. I kept all the extra weight for over three years but I didn't smoke.

During my withdrawal I felt like a robot. Even my lips felt numb. I didn't feel real emotional because I kept eating lots of ice cream and other sweets. Eating kept me in a state of "drunkenness" or "nicotineness." I was truly in a daze and actually walked into a couple walls. I was really out of it. I would forget why I was having such a hard time or why I seemed to be so dazed. Friends reminded me that I'd just quit smoking. It didn't make sense to me but I trusted them that I was going through withdrawal. After about six weeks I went to a chiropractor who recommended a lot of vitamins, particularly vitamin C. Vitamin C helped get rid of some of the toxins in my system. He promised I'd already been through the worst of it, and I started taking a lot of vitamin C.

I began feeling very proud that I had quit smoking. Having my cough go away almost immediately was a great benefit. Having the freedom to not check every minute if I had cigarettes and matches and everything that I used to have to carry around with me was the best of all. I never carried just one pack; I carried two packs in case I'd smoke the first pack. The feeling of freedom was great. It made me happy to see how thrilled my children were that I was a non-smoker.

I've really struggled with the weight gain and I even considered smoking again, but I know what addiction is and I know that if I even smoke one cigarette, I may not be able to give them up again. I know if I ever give in, I will be done. The hardest times for me are when I'm walking into the house where I live as a sorority house mother and I see a single cigarette laying on the floor. I want to pick it up and smoke it. I don't know why. It's just that a cigarette in its purest state really tempts me.

For me the best part of not smoking has been the knowledge that I'm no longer doing something that is abusive, unhealthy, and a dirty habit. I love myself enough to go through whatever I have to go through to be good to myself. I feel sad when I look at smokers, when I realize what they're doing and how hard it is for them to quit. I wish I could give them something to help them get off cigarettes. What I've noticed about women who smoke is that their skin color is generally gray. They just look less healthy than non-smokers.

I realize now that smoking smells awful. I didn't realize how bad I had smelled until I quit. My clothes smelled so bad. My kids used to tell me that and I didn't believe them because I couldn't smell anything. After I stopped smoking, I couldn't believe how bad my closet smelled. It was like a heavily used ashtray.

As I look back on my life, I realize that in order to stay sober, I had to get out of my marriage and I guess I thought if I could get out of that marriage, with all the pain that entailed, then I could quit smoking. Now I'm into physical fitness. I can feel the difference when I don't exercise. I begin to notice a feeling of lethargy or depression settling in if I don't get enough exercise.

The most important thing I realized in the process of quitting smoking was that it wasn't as hard as I had expected. It was all the negative self-talk before quitting that had convinced me I couldn't make it. There are a lot of other things that I have done in the past eight years that were much harder and much more painful than quitting smoking.

MATT

Age 45. Retired commercial airline pilot; married, no children; works full-time as a hobbyist building vintage cars, cabins, and furniture for his and his wife's personal use.

I started smoking leaves when I was about nine years old. In the fall we would take the leaves that fell off the oak trees and roll them in newspapers to make cigars. We'd wet the leaves down and roll them up in our hands to get them into small pieces. Then we'd roll them in a dampened newspaper. They would actually look like cigars. And because I was really good with my hands, I got to be the best cigar maker in the neighborhood. I used to have a cigar box full of leaf and newspaper cigars and all the boys would come to my tent and we would smoke these every fall. It was a tradition that lasted for two or three years. It was a wonderful fall ritual.

When I got into high school, due to peer pressure, I started smoking real cigarettes with a bunch of kids I rode to school with. At about sixteen or seventeen, my folks said, "If you're going to smoke, you might as well smoke at home." So I started smoking at home when I was in high school, about 1957 or 1958. My folks never discussed whether smoking was good or bad. It was a grown-up's habit. My folks had always said that it would stunt a person's growth. I don't know where that notion came from but it was a popular one in those years.

I was used to being around smokers. My dad smoked moderate to heavy. My mom smoked light to moderate, and all of my aunts, uncles, and cousins who were adults smoked. Someone who didn't smoke was the exception in my family.

I loved smoking when I was a young kid. It made me feel grown-up. It made me feel like I'd reached manhood or adulthood because only adults could do it. I had the feeling of being accepted. The only two times I felt really accepted as an adult by my parents was when they said I could drive the car and smoke cigarettes in the house. Smoking was a major rite of passage into adulthood. I even liked the yellow stains on my fingers. They were a badge or a mark of status. They proved I wasn't smoking Kents. A real man smoked a Camel or a Lucky. In my mind, there were real men's cigarettes and then there were women's cigarettes. I would smoke three or four Camels and let them burn down on my hand until it hurt. That made my fingers dark brown. I can remember a friend's dad who was a welder and a real tough guy. He had serious brown stains between the first and second fingers on his hand. That impressed me. He was a real man. The smell, and taste, and the burns all seemed attractive at the time.

I went into the Navy out of high school and there it was standard procedure to smoke. There were designated times and places where we could smoke and they just automatically assumed and joked that the only reason you wouldn't smoke is that you were out of a designated area. During my military years I smoked a pack a day maybe. I probably stayed at a pack a day for the next five years.

In the early to the mid-sixties, the Surgeon General informed the public that smoking was not good for us. At the same time, I started flying airplanes. I was involved with a different group of people than in the military or in college. These people were more concerned about their medical performance and their ability to pass medical exams every six months. I was getting the message that smoking was not healthy. I was starting to fly and going to moderately high altitudes of 15,000 to 18,000 feet. I was flying in the mountains and doing work with the forest service without oxygen on board and I was getting dull headaches. I talked to several people about it and deduced that my headaches were caused by the smoking. I'd go up in altitude for three hours at 15,000 or 16,000 feet, smoke half-a-dozen cigarettes, and come down with a dull headache. I believed it was from oxygen starvation, so I started chewing tobacco and I developed a fairly strong habit almost immediately.

I went from cigarettes to leaf chewing tobacco and within months I was a serious Copenhagen user. I found that by chewing I could get my nicotine fix not only stronger and easier but steadily, all the time, even when my hands were busy. When I smoked, I couldn't feed my nicotine habit when I was busy with my hands. I immediately became real interested in chewing and increased the doses. I didn't spit. I swallowed the nicotine. I felt spitting was pretty socially unacceptable so I swallowed the saliva. I figured real men did it that way. Only the wimps spit out the juice. Of course, that meant I was not only taking that much nicotine in my mouth but in my stomach too. I was getting very heavy doses of nicotine and I developed a heavy habit that lasted 20 or 21 years.

I got more conscious of the health risks and, because I had to take a medical test every year, I realized that if I wanted to pass the exams, smoking was not a good deal. It was harmful. For twenty years I knew I shouldn't be doing tobacco of any kind. However, I believed that smoking was more harmful than chewing. I was deluded about Copenhagen. For ten or twelve years I pretended that Copenhagen wasn't that harmful because it wasn't damaging my lungs.

During my early years on Copenhagen, not too much was known about its health consequences. But about ten years ago, I started hearing things about mouth cancer. The mouth is a much more efficient organ. Sucking on Copenhagen means taking it directly into the bloodstream. I gradually became more aware of the damage I was doing and I started suffering headaches too. I felt like there was a connection between my headaches and the nicotine poison in my body.

For about ten years I tried to quit Copenhagen and when I didn't have a can of Copenhagen, I smoked cigarettes if they were available. Sometimes I would even do both. Sometimes I would have Copenhagen in my mouth and if we were sitting around the table drinking coffee and someone was smoking a cigarette, I would smoke a cigarette too because it was fun to do. But by the late seventies, and early eighties, it was so socially unacceptable that I quit doing cigarettes altogether. I felt like anybody who did cigarettes in public was really thought of as a fool. I looked down on people who did cigarettes as weak and foolish. My tobacco use was not a public thing, and if someone caught me doing cigarettes, I felt embarrassed.

I have a whole history of quitting. I would quit doing tobacco altogether, everything; no cigarettes, no chewing tobacco of any sort. I'd put on ten or twelve pounds within a period of six months or less because of my oral fixation. I would suck on lots of candy and eat lots of desserts and too much food. I knew I could lose the weight immediately if I started chewing tobacco again, so I would, automatically and deliberately. I did that many times during a period of ten years. And yet I was in a lot of denial. I didn't consciously feel like I was doing suicide on the installment plan. I deliberately denied that there was any problem with my tobacco use. I could quit anytime! I'd prove it! I would just do it for a few days or a few weeks. It was not going to be a big problem. And then every once in awhile reality would hit me in my face. I'd look back and realize I'd been doing tobacco again for three or four years.

I got into recovery from alcoholism, and the

treatment process taught me how to confront reality. I started looking at this issue and knew I shouldn't be doing it. I knew I was killing myself and when I kept on doing it I'd hate myself. The only way to live with myself was to either quit or deny. I did one or the other for ten years.

I began to really get in trouble with my values. I would quit and then become a closet user so my wife wouldn't know. I would hide my supply. I could do that for up to six months before she caught me. And it was real painful. I was embarrassed and ashamed because I knew that I didn't want to do it. I knew that I had implied or directly told her that I didn't want her to help me. So when I was doing it, I knew that she would be real disappointed. It was real shameful.

This last quitting feels different. My dad got cancer of the throat. He was a heavy smoker for 50 years, and then got cancer of the throat at age 75. It started with just a cough he couldn't get rid of. He went to the doctor, and by the time they diagnosed it, it was necessary to take his larynx. They were able to salvage enough of his voice box so that he could kind of make himself understood, but having gone through that process with him and being there at the hospital every day or so for weeks on end and seeing all these people at the hospital with their voice boxes gone really shook me. The guy in the bed next to my dad was a Copenhagen user and he had part of his chin cut off and his lower jaw cut away. They grafted a bone from his leg to his face.

That experience really forced me to confront

the issue of heredity and the suicide and my own use — all those things that I'd been denying for years. I came to the realization that I don't have the choice anymore of choosing to do it. I can't choose it anymore. My belief in heredity is strong enough that I don't have that choice to use tobacco. I'm confronted with facts about heredity that I believe in.

Each time I've quit, my process has been to have a date that had a meaningful connection. I've used the first of January, or my birthday, or Labor Day. I believed that I needed a date to quit that had some significance. This last time, I quit on my sister's and mother's birthday, the thirteenth of June.

The first two weeks I went into a rage on two separate occasions. One was with one of my very best friends and it was over something totally insignificant. As far as our relationship was concerned, it was a totally needless point. And I flew into a rage that went on for days. About a week or ten days later, I saw him again and as we tried to discuss it, I flew into another rage that went on for several hours. My wife helped me see how out of control I was with rage, and I began to connect the fact that I was using tobacco to get me through periods of time when I needed to deal with my feelings. But instead, I would take a hit of tobacco and stuff the feelings down. I'd use tobacco like a drug. Instead of saying, "I'm really feeling angry," I would just take a hit of tobacco and not do anything with the rage. I had a lot of rage over a lot of things that I was stuffing.

During that first two weeks my feelings were acutely apparent. I haven't had any rageful episodes since the first two weeks and I've got three or four months off tobacco.

I was heavily addicted. I think cigarettes are pretty mild in comparison to Copenhagen. Cigarettes are diluted with oxygen as you draw them in. There's only so much nicotine that can be absorbed, even when you're a chain-smoker sixteen or eighteen hours a day. I was getting more nicotine in my blood by not spitting and having tobacco in my mouth every single waking moment of the day, except those three meals of fifteen minutes or whatever they were. Sometimes I even slept with Copenhagen in my mouth so I kept getting a good supply into my bloodstream.

When I finally got off, I had a withdrawal similar to the withdrawal from heroin, an itchiness that felt like it was from within. I'd scratch but it wouldn't relieve it. The itchiness was all over my entire body. It went on four or five days and nights. I was most acutely aware of it at night. I would wake up every fifteen or twenty minutes and scratch all over my body; scratch my head, shoulders, legs, chest, and torso. I'd itch from within but I would scratch from without. I wouldn't be able to relieve the itching. It was a mildly uncomfortable itch that would keep me awake. Then I would fall back to sleep and wake up in twenty minutes and do it again.

To help me over my urges to use again, I used the Alcoholics Anonymous program of one day at a time. I don't have to quit forever; I can go back

118

and use tobacco tomorrow if I want to. All I have to do is just not use it today. Someone asked me one day how many years I'd been using Copenhagen. I said, "A few years, maybe five." I stopped and added it up and it was 21 years. That's 21 years of one day at a time. It seemed like five. So why couldn't the reverse be true? I could be off tobacco for 21 years but it may seem like a couple years; or I could be off for a couple years but it may seem like just a couple months. In other words, I can put that shrinkage of time to my benefit. I don't have to quit forever or one year or five years or twenty. Just one day is all I have to quit for and they'll add up. One day someone will say, "How long have you been off cigarettes or off tobacco?" and I'll say, "Oh, I don't know, a few years." And I'll sit down and add it up and discover it's been 21 years.

Like the earlier times when I quit, I feared putting on weight. So I made a decision to start exercising on a regular basis. And because I was getting on to mid-age and because of my father's arthritic condition and my own indications of the onset of arthritis, I decided to begin a serious and regular exercise program. Again, I made the decision to not do it forever, but to just do it for a short period of time. I would do it without question and without reneging on that promise. My initial promise to myself to exercise was for a period of six months. No matter what, I would do it for an hour three days a week, and then I would reassess. At that time, I would have a chance to see if I'd put on extra weight. And if I had, I would make another choice to either go back to tobacco or to increase my exercise or to decrease my caloric intake.

Since quitting I've felt like I'm in a honeymoon period. I'm real positive. Physically I've felt real strong. The arthritis that used to bother me in the mornings hasn't been there for the last couple months. I don't know if it's the exercise or the fact that I haven't got those poisons running through my bloodstream anymore or both. I just feel a lot more positive, a lot better about myself.

I miss the tobacco. I think of it as a wonderful friend. It offered solace from pain. It was a wonderful way to retreat from it. For years I had used drugs to hide from pain, whether emotional, physical, or mental. I still think of tobacco every day even though I'm happier not using it. But it's like any addiction. This is no different in my mind. Nicotine is a drug, and I'm an addictive personality. I look at the drug as one of my best friends, and I know that I'm only one cigarette away from being back to a two-pack-a-day user. But I can't afford the luxury of doing it. It's a friend that I really know is an enemy. It's one of my worst enemies that I think of as a friend. It's the great paradox that alcohol and other drugs have played in people's lives. They think of drugs as friends because they can retreat from their pain. People do it for many, many years and all of a sudden find out they can't do it anymore. The friend has turned into an enemy. That's how I think of tobacco.

That friend, after all those years, is now one of

my worst enemies. He tried to kill me and I became conscious of that change in our friendship. I don't know why. I guess my own perception changed. Maybe it was a miracle. For many years I was privy to all the facts about tobacco as a killer but I still chose to deny them. I don't know why at this time I think of it as one of my worst enemies. I just know I don't have the luxury of making friends because this person will kill me.

I grieve for smokers because I know there's nothing I can say or do that will change them from smoking or chewing or whatever it is they do. I know they have to change in their own time and with their own process. All I can do is not smoke. Maybe my example will help someone else.

I've learned that a drug is a drug. It's suicide on the installment plan for an addictive personality like mine. No longer killing myself on an installment plan feels wonderful. I feel like I'm voting to live rather than voting to die. I'm enjoying life enough to want to stay alive for it. Even though that's how I feel, I still think about tobacco every day but I just say to myself, "Don't do it today. Just chew some gum, or eat some candy — just don't do it today."

As the months and years go by, I know I'll think about it less often. But even if I never get over the urge, I just hope I can remember that all I've got to do is not do it for twenty more minutes. That's all I've got to worry about.

TERRY

Age 40. Professional writer and editor; married, father of two boys; loves humor, playing baseball, and the Chicago Cubs.

Neither I nor most of my friends in the early years smoked. They were either athletes or at least into athletics of some kind. It was obvious the ones who did smoke. They were always short of wind.

We hadn't smoked because of school rules around athletics. It was just the way we played in grade school. When I reached high school, there were rules that no student could smoke, but of course anybody who wanted to did. And they did, all over the grounds. I had some friends who smoked in high school but it just never occurred to me to smoke.

I was slow in taking to smoking and I didn't take to it much even when I was in college. I remember one occasion during my sophomore year. I was feeling really lost. I think I was in college to please my folks more than myself. I got into sitting up all night in the dorm rooms, talking to my buddies in all-night conversations and one of them smoked. One night I decided I'd try a cigarette. I smoked a few Tareytons and they tasted awful. And I thought, oh boy, how can anybody do this? My friend said, "Hey, that's okay. Don't judge it on one night; you'll get used to it." However, I went out the next morning and bought a pack of L&Ms instead.

I smoked a couple and noticed that they did funny things when you lit them. Sometimes there'd be a little explosion on the end of the cigarette. One side would burn and the other side wouldn't. I thought, wow, what is this stuff? I tossed them and I didn't smoke again until the next fall when I bought a different kind. Even then, I bought cigarettes only once in awhile. I might buy a pack on a Friday if I had money and I'd smoke one every once in awhile until they were gone. It was usually an occasional thing. Smoking was a reward if I finished a paper or maybe a test.

In the spring of my junior year, I was very tense again. I didn't know if I wanted to stay in school and I started cutting class. At the same time, I ran out of money, so I wasn't smoking. I dropped out of school and it took me a couple months to get a job. After I started working, I would have a cigarette every once in awhile. There was something about smoking and taking a break. One of the people I worked with smoked, and he took a break in the morning and a break in the afternoon. I'd take cigarettes to work and leave them in my desk drawer and have a cigarette on break. And then at night, if I was going out, I would take two or three out of the pack to take along. But I still wasn't really into smoking. I don't think I was addicted to the nicotine although I really liked the effect of it. I had realized the first night that I smoked, years earlier, that after I had one, I didn't feel the next three or four that I had. I wasn't sure why that was the case, but smoking energized me. The nicotine made me tremble and it made me high.

Shortly thereafter, in February of 1966, I got drafted. There was a lot going on in my life at that point and I was not yet 21. I wished I was a heavy smoker. I wished I was short of breath and had spots on my lungs so they wouldn't take me. Before they drafted me I had still been smoking but not much. Usually I just couldn't afford it. I could barely afford to live. At that time my big indulgence was going down to Mr. Steak on Sunday afternoon or sometimes I'd go for a pizza.

In basic training we couldn't have anything, no personal possessions. The only thing we could buy was cigarettes. Everybody smoked and so did I. I smoked nonfiltered cigarettes because if we smoked filters, we had to keep the leftover filters in our pockets when we were done with a cigarette. We couldn't just drop them on the ground. We had to "fieldstrip" all butts, which meant let all the tobacco out and roll the paper up in a tiny little ball and keep that in our pocket. The idea was to keep the ground clean. This training was also to protect us in combat. If we were in combat and we camped some place, nothing could be left behind that would leave a trace. The army was real strict about smoking.

After not smoking much for years, I was all of a sudden smoking unfiltered Pall Malls and, even today, I can't look at a pack of Pall Malls without thinking of basic training. That was the only time I ever smoked them. I must have smoked two or three cartons during basic training. There was nothing else to do and it kept me occupied. It was a cheap activity. Cigarettes were only fifteen cents a pack. It was better than going to the PX and drinking 3.2 beer. Smoking was something I could do. I would sit out on the fire escape and I felt like the actor Robert Taylor, who really knew how to smoke a cigarette. It was kind of dramatic to sit out there on the fire escape and light up with the sun going down. My real history with smoking started then, and I smoked all through the Army.

And then in 1969, about a year after I got out of the Army, I quit. I decided I just didn't want to smoke anymore. I had gotten married and gone back to school. The first year I was back in school, we were pretty poor. We lived on the GI Bill which wasn't a lot of money. I wasn't eating enough and my weight was down to about 155 pounds. I figured if I stopped smoking, we'd have more money for food. It was a real simple equation. So I quit and immediately my taste buds came back. I started getting hungry and I ate a lot more food. I was afraid I was going to get fat so I started working out with weights and riding a bicycle everywhere. I put on about twenty pounds but it was good weight. And then about a year after I quit, my wife quit. Neither of us smoked for the rest of the time we were in undergraduate school in Illinois.

We went from there to the writers' program in Iowa City, Iowa. My wife moved to Iowa City before me because I had three weeks left to work and we needed to save all the money we could. I moved her into our new apartment and returned to Illinois and worked the three weeks. When I got back to Iowa, she was smoking again. That bummed me out but I didn't say anything. Almost two years later, I started bumming cigarettes from her once in awhile. Occasionally I'd have a cigarette if I really felt like having one. And that seemed okay. It was a positive decision. But then I started smoking regularly again and I was looking to feel the effects. I wanted that sensation I'd gotten years before. Otherwise smoking was just a habit with no reward.

From then on I smoked until I quit three years ago. There were some brief periods when I didn't smoke. Some summers I didn't because I was playing softball. I didn't want to carry cigarettes around with me and I didn't want smoking to affect my wind. They were a lot of trouble. They'd spill out of the pack in my bag and get all over and be ruined. If I really wanted to have one, I'd borrow one, but, of course, nobody likes someone who does that. Finally, three years ago, I quit.

One of the things that encouraged it was that I was sharing an office with a smoker and the room got awfully smoky, so smoky that even I didn't like it. D-Day came around and I thought I'd try not smoking. I figured I'd quit and get healthier. At the time, I was thinking about changing my life a lot, quitting a lot of things, like not playing kids' games anymore. I was nearly 40 and figured I needed to spend more time doing yard work than playing softball. And

I decided quitting smoking was another change I needed to make. So I did.

I didn't think about quitting ahead of time. I made no preparation for it. The first time that I had quit years earlier, somebody had suggested I smoke one less cigarette each day. And I figured, why bother? That just makes it harder because you think about it. I knew it would be easier for me to just stop.

That first day I didn't have an urge to have a cigarette until after I ate lunch. And the urge lasted about half a minute. A friend had suggested I try lemon drops to satisfy the urge. I bought lemon drops and had one. I learned the first time I quit that nicotine was a blood sugar and that without cigarettes I craved sweets more, including soda. This time I got into yogurt, too, the kind with fruit. I quite literally replaced cigarettes with sugar for a while.

I didn't really have any physical withdrawal from smoking. I just had the urge that would come up once in awhile. I also had a flat dry feeling in my mouth. But a drink of water made it go away. Even though I haven't had a cigarette for three years, I do like to have a cigar once in awhile. It's a ritual and it has to do with my past. My grandpa smoked cigars when he'd sit around with the boys. So when my brother, Dave, and I sit around, we'll have a cigar occasionally. Dave doesn't smoke cigarettes either.

Quitting, for me, was not physically difficult, but quitting any activity that rewards us means losing something from your life. During the early period of not smoking three years ago, when I thought of smoking as an unpleasant activity, it was easy not to do it. But when I'd remember smoking as associated with pleasant times, like sitting around after dinner with friends, then it was difficult. I knew something was missing. It wasn't the same to go get a lemon drop and rejoin the group at the dinner table. And it wasn't as romantic a feeling to sit around on the porch at sunset and suck on a lemon drop, so "Robert Taylor" was gone.

I'm aware too that smoking provides something for the fingers to do. Often I wanted to have a cigarette because I was in a special situation where I didn't know what to do with my hands. With smoking it's an automatic thing. You have an occupation for your hands. You move your hand from your mouth to the ashtray. It's rehearsed. There's a certain protocol. It's probably akin to the proper way one stood with hands in pockets in the eighteenth century.

As a smoker, there were things "preordained" for me to do with my hands. After quitting, there were times when I wished I had a cigarette, but I'd think about something else and drink a glass of water. I discovered a glass of water was a real good substitute because I'd hold it in my hand and move it to my mouth. It's almost the same kind of hand to mouth activity as smoking. And it's good for you. I hardly ever drank water before even though I knew I needed lots of water every day. So for me to drink water was cleansing. I used to image swallowing it, and watching it travel throughout my system. It only took a little while to get over the urge to smoke. Even if I thought about the cigarette for more than a minute, the sensation would go away. Even if I tried to keep that sensation, it would go away. I think something in the body happens and if you don't gratify the sensation, it just goes away.

I'm satisfied that I'm no longer gratifying the urge for a cigarette. I like not being dependent on cigarettes. However, smoking a cigar once in awhile disqualifies me from being a total non-smoker. Cigarettes are real hard to get out of your system. I do think there's an addiction at work and maybe I've replaced it with something else. I'm not sure. But I am sure that living free of cigarettes gives me more energy. That's the number one benefit, having more mental and more physical energy. I have more willingness and more time to do other things. If a person smokes a pack a day and it takes seven minutes to smoke a cigarette, that's 140 minutes a day, almost two and a half hours spent smoking rather than doing something productive. People write books in that amount of time.

Another benefit of not smoking is having more money. A pack of cigarettes costs more than a dollar. Maybe even a buck-and-a-half; that's ten dollars a week. With forty dollars a month I can buy needed clothes or make a monthly payment to buy a word processor. The money adds up and that's like anything else, it's done a little bit at a time. Energy, money, and, of course, the bottom line is health — three great benefits.

It's kind of nice thinking it might be different for my kids. My dad smoked and both my grandfathers smoked. It was the manly thing to do for me. Everybody smoked on television and everybody smoked in the movies. And they don't do that much anymore. You hardly ever see somebody smoke on television or in the movies, and the kids get training in school. My son came home the other day and lectured his mother, who still smokes, about what happens to your heart when you inhale. Everything constricts in your heart. He had the whole thing down that he'd learned in his health class. It was about blood circulation but they talked about smoking and I'm sure that smoking will be part of every organ system they study in school. A subtle message is there that isn't so subtle after all and I don't think my kids will smoke.

I think a good way to stop smoking, if someone wants to try, is to make a promise to yourself to stop for the next hour and see how easy it is. You can do it an hour at a time that way. Just get a clean glass and stand by the sink if you have to. You find that you must fill that time. You're not going to avoid the urge that is crying for a cigarette. So you sweep the kitchen floor or change the oil in the car. Just do something. But if it's possible to stop for an hour, then it's possible to stop for good. And everybody stops for an hour, unless they don't sleep. Everybody becomes a nonsmoker in his or her sleep.

CONNIE

*Age 36. A human resources profes-
sional occupationally; a mountain
climber and tournament squash
player by avocation; also loves her
new Victorian home, saunas, and
good books.*

I began smoking when I was twelve or thirteen. Every day, I walked to school with three
girls who were a year older, and we'd stop in the
park so they could have a cigarette on the way. It
wasn't long until I wanted to be like them and
have a cigarette too. My parents would have
thought it was uncool, definitely. I'd leave for
school about ten minutes before my sister even
though we'd both be going to the same school
and walking the same route. It was a little per-
plexing to my family that I'd leave ten minutes
before her, but to smoke with my friends, I had
to. None of us kids were allowed to smoke at
home.

I didn't really become a regular smoker, smoking heavily, until on vacation in high school. We
were restricted at school and many of my activities didn't allow me to smoke. But by the time I
went to college, I had full freedom and I was
smoking a lot. However, "a lot" in those days
wasn't as much as it was later for me.

Interestingly enough, I had a few friends who
were smoking then but I always hung out with a
physically active crowd and many of them didn't
smoke. That was a major hurdle. Philosophically,

131

smoking presented me with a conflict. My first boyfriend in college was a downhill skier and he hated smoking. He was so disgusted with it that I had to use mouthwash before he would kiss me. I was so stubborn about my smoking. However, it started to wear on me, even then, because it really did not fit with what I valued. It was awkward for me to smoke because of the things I liked to do. For instance, it was awkward to smoke while riding a chair lift.

But I kept smoking and sometime later I applied to be an instructor at the Minnesota Outward Bound School. The guy was coming out to interview me at my home and I'd never met him before. I'd warned my roommate not to talk about smoking. I wanted to impress him and show him that I could really do this job. We set up the house to make it look outdoorsy. My hiking boots were near the door. He said, "Let's go to a Chinese restaurant. I hear there's one nearby." I called up to my roommate to see if she knew where it was and she said, "Oh yes, that's where you bought the pack of cigarettes the other day." I about died. That blew my cover but I got the job anyway. That was my junior year; it was 1971. I worked there that summer and I didn't smoke openly, but I snuck around to smoke. I kept it hidden for three months and I thought I was getting away with it. Of course, now I realize that when you're 30 days in the woods, everyone knows what's going on, so they knew I was sneaking smokes, but I thought I was hiding it. Besides, I'm sure they smelled it on me.

Many years later I started going out with another man who I didn't want to smoke in front of. By this time, I was in such conflict over smoking that I decided I wasn't going to smoke in front of him. We went out a few times and I didn't smoke. But I couldn't maintain it. One night, when we were out for dinner, I told him I smoked. He had known it all along. Nobody is ever really fooled.

I had good preparation for smoking from childhood on because I grew up in a smoking setting. My parents both smoked but they stopped. My mother says her quitting was almost a religious experience. And my father stopped by using a "one day at a time theory." He still says he just does not smoke right now. He more or less used the A.A. "one day at a time" philosophy without knowing anything about A.A. My siblings and I all smoked but I was the die-hard smoker. I was the most obviously addicted one in the family. I smoked the most and I was the least open about it. Also, I was the first one to stop. My brother has now stopped too, so we have two down, three to go. But I had continued smoking for years even though it interfered with my value system.

In 1980 I went on an expedition to Mt. McKinley in Alaska. I didn't smoke cigarettes during my twelve weeks of training. But I smoked a pipe. Philosophically, it seemed acceptable to pull out the pipe. There I was, dying from the strain, skiing up to the base of Mt. McKinley and yet preoccupied with smoking. I never got off nicotine during that time. Even though I didn't smoke cigarettes, I got my nicotine and that was a true pleasure. That was one of life's small pleasures during that time. Not smoking cigarettes was a big thing for me.

Smoking had such importance that it got in the way of a lot of my activities. I remember packing to go on a six-day mountain climb and carefully packing my cigarettes. I ignored the paradox. I remember many trips with Outward Bound, twelve-day backpacking trips and carrying enough cigarettes to last throughout the trip. I would take enough for me and then if there was someone else along who was starting to borrow cigarettes, I'd guard my stash. There was no way I could get another supply where I was. I remember one trip when I had misjudged my rations, or maybe I'd lost a couple of packs in the water or something. I rationed myself three a day, taking only a hit off one occasionally. Then I would tap it out just to make sure I never was without.

I really didn't like my cigarette habit. I was ashamed a lot because of my activities. Most people were really surprised that I smoked. I was self-conscious about it. Many people have told me I was a very respectful smoker. Because I really didn't want people to remember that I smoked, I was very conscious of where my smoke was going. For instance, if I was on a camping or backpacking trip, I would only smoke around the campfire in the evening when people wouldn't notice it so much. I was hiding it and trying to be subtle about it, trying to be inconspicuous from

134

almost day one. I was open about my smoking only at a big party or something where a lot of people were smoking.

I first began thinking of quitting smoking before I was twenty. Mom and Dad said that they would pay us children if we stopped smoking by the time we were 21. But I didn't. The Mt. McKinley trip got me thinking about it but I decided that going on the trip was big enough. Quitting crossed my mind a lot but I didn't do much about it although I started asking others who had stopped, how they'd stopped. I loved hearing other people's stories about how they stopped. I was curious about it because I knew I wanted to stop someday. I talked about stopping smoking but not about *me* stopping smoking. I got literature and I read articles and the ads about stop-smoking programs. I never went to any of them but I always read about them with interest, and I began to cut the articles out.

Then my brother went to a hypnotist in New York to quit smoking. I was living in New York, too, and he and I were together right after his visit to the hypnotist. He was so calm and he simply stopped smoking. I was really impressed. I referred another friend of mine to a hypnotist and he stopped too. I thought, wow, this must really be something else. By this time I'd moved from New York but I made an appointment with the hypnotist and flew back there, ostensibly to visit friends, but my real reason was to go to see the hypnotist. I didn't tell anybody what I was doing except the people I was visiting in Connecticut. I

135

wanted a cigarette so bad. But I did go to the hypnotist and I got the tape of what he'd said. However, I knew it didn't feel right when I left that Friday. His process was to ask me why I wanted to stop, what I didn't like about smoking, and what I was doing there. During the hypnosis, he repeated back exactly what I'd told him: Smoking was a value conflict for me. I really liked the act of smoking but because I valued my health, and I liked physical exercise, smoking got in my way. My lungs hurt a lot during some of my activities and I was embarrassed that I smoked. It didn't fit with my own self-image. But I stopped for only two days. I bought a little tape recorder to listen to the tapes he gave me, but they didn't help. The second I left my friend's house, I went straight to the train station and got a pack of cigarettes. I kept that experience my little secret. But I don't chastise myself at all for that and I don't chastise other people for their attempts to stop. I think that's all part of being ready. I made no other real attempts to stop.

I liked smoking, I liked the ritual to it. I associated smoking with slowing down; it felt calming, soothing a little bit. I liked the taste, except I didn't like what it meant. And yet sitting around, talking on the telephone, and having cigarettes and coffee was a pretty nice way to spend a couple of hours.

Even though for years I pretended I smoked only a pack a day, I'm sure I smoked at least two packs a day. And as I started thinking about stopping, I actually smoked more because I knew that I was going to be stopping. I always had a carton around.

When I really got serious about stopping, I talked to a lot of people to get ideas. I remember a conversation that really hit me. I was with a friend in a restaurant. She said rather than feel deprived by quitting, become a nonsmoker instead. That was similar to how my father had done it. It made more sense to me then than it had twenty years earlier when my dad did it.

There wasn't any event in my life to prepare me like a horrible cancer story. I had thought about stopping on D-Day; although I didn't dare say to anyone that I was planning to actually stop on D-Day, I did commit myself to not smoking on that day. A friend at work asked me if he could use me to advertise D-Day in an article for the company newsletter. His article implied that I might be thinking about quitting for a longer term than just one day and I was really ticked off at him. I wasn't planning to do that.

Before D-Day I decided I wanted to do everything to stack the cards to my advantage. So I dusted off my hypnosis tapes. I bought another self-help tape so I had two hypnosis tapes. And I got Nicorette gum. I remember being high, sort of excited, wound up, full of high energy that first day. And the stopping lasted longer than D-Day. I made myself listen to that tape twice a day, come hell or high water. And I did not let other things get in the way. I'm usually not quite that disciplined but I was very disciplined about the tapes. Not smoking was my top priority and I

137

really pushed myself to keep it there. I chewed the gum and I didn't apologize for that. I wrestled with doing the gum because I knew it was nicotine. I think a placebo might have worked just as well. I chewed two or three pieces a day for a couple months. I got mouth sores and they're really awful. I weaned myself from the gum. I got down to chewing one piece a day. I set a deadline for myself and I quit. I actually had two or three pieces of gum left but I decided I didn't want to do it anymore.

After quitting, I gained weight. My appetite really increased. Someone had said that grapefruit would clear the nicotine out of my system faster. And I ate a lot of grapefruit and drank grapefruit juice. I really believe it helped. I never ate so much grapefruit as I did in those first few days. With as much fruit as I ate, it's no wonder my mouth was sore.

I exercised a little bit more, too, after quitting. I did that almost as a substitute. I wanted to feel the positive effects of not smoking so I increased my exercise program. Surprisingly enough, it didn't feel as good as fast as I would have expected. In spite of smoking for twenty-some years, I thought that one week after stopping, I'd feel much better out on the squash court, but it really didn't work that way. I was very fascinated about what might be happening with my body, so I started reading some articles. I wanted to learn how long it would take for my lungs to regenerate. It takes five to ten years to replace the tissue if you smoked as long as I did. I've got a ways to go before my body is totally cleansed but it's well on its way to being cleansed.

Emotionally it wasn't that difficult for me to stop. I was really ready. I didn't want to be a smoker anymore. And I developed a little theory that I call the 51 percent theory. Fifty-one percent of me wanted to be a nonsmoker. And as long as the ratio was 51 to 49, I wouldn't smoke. I still wanted to smoke but I mentally pictured these two little bodies inside my stomach that would go to battle whenever I wanted a cigarette, and the 51 percent body kept overthrowing the other one. These two cartoon characters fought it out many times and the 51 percent character always won. Whenever I wanted a cigarette, I just closed my eyes and said, "Now, you two deal with it." It was important that more of me wanted to be not smoking than smoking. That made all the difference. I believe that when you're ready to quit, when the time is right, then it isn't that much of a struggle. I really wanted not to smoke again.

I love the freedom of not smoking. I feel so much freer, going places, being with people. Smoking really ruled me more than I'd like to admit. It really controlled what I would do and wouldn't do — like running, for instance. I knew I could never be a serious runner and smoke. I run now although I'm still not a serious runner. But it isn't an absurdity to think I could actually, *really* run. The same with other sports. I can really go ahead and do what I want with activities and I don't have a struggle with smoking. When

I joined the squash club, I was the only one who would come out after a game and light a cigarette.

Other things have changed too. One day a co-worker asked if I'd like to ride with him to a meeting. I knew I'd have to be in the car for an hour not smoking, so I said no. I was bothered by meetings and movies, times when you knew you were going to have a block of time when you couldn't smoke. I was always aware of that and now I'm free. The freedom is the biggest benefit of not smoking. I feel much better physically even though I have gained weight. I decided early on I wasn't going to let the weight gain bother me too much because I think it will adjust itself over time. It hasn't been quite a year and I've stabilized. I don't feel like I'm gaining anymore. I think I've hit the top of the pyramid and now I'm on the downside.

It's wonderful not being in conflict with my values anymore. I think quitting is the best thing I've ever done for myself. Smoking had haunted me since the early 1970s. When I first stopped smoking, I was a little hesitant to talk much about it because I didn't trust I'd be able to follow through with it. But I had a couple key friends who knew I was doing it, and that was good because I needed support. I couldn't talk with my parents about it much, even though they'd stopped, because I wasn't sure I could go through with it. Mostly I was quiet about it.

I have not become a self-righteous nonsmoker. I hated it when someone was self-righteous around me. I try to be empathetic towards smokers because I know that they probably don't like the fact that they're smoking. However, it does bother me a bit. I hate being in a car with all the windows closed with a smoker.

I've come to believe that if people want to quit, they should allow themselves to celebrate not smoking. They should see it as a choice, and see it as something they want to do for themselves. They should give themselves permission to eat a little more. They shouldn't beat-up on themselves if they don't do it right the first time, but think of it as a step in the right direction.

Something that helped me gain strength was that I literally looked at myself in the mirror more than once and said, "You are a nonsmoker and you want to stay that way." I did a lot of self-talk. That and the 51 percent theory gave me strength. Relying on these two tools meant I didn't have to deal with the urge anymore. I turned it over to these two little voices and I didn't have to struggle with wanting a cigarette for very long. Another thing I did was pamper myself. I took saunas, and put two dollars away every day in a straw basket to spend on something I really wanted. After a few weeks of saving, I took my 65 or 70 dollars, bought myself a world map and had it mounted. And that world map to this day is very special because it's connected to the new me. I also treated myself to things like *Glamour* or *Vogue* magazine. I usually never spent money on things like that.

I did worry, at first, about my productivity. I

was an early riser and always smoked, drank coffee, and did good work real early in the morning before going to my job. And I can't do that anymore. That bothers me some but it's not worth going back to smoking for. There is nothing that I can think of that would be worth my starting again. I think I'm a lifer. I get a little worried saying that because it's only been a year but I don't want to smoke again. I really don't want to smoke again. And I think I'm free.

TIM

Age 34. Married; computer buff; excels in management; well-read in current affairs; loves photography, mind games, and good conversation.

I decided when I was in high school that I would not smoke because it wasn't good for me. I remember getting lectured about smoking by a couple of older guys who used to lifeguard. And most of my friends didn't smoke. Since there was a group of us who didn't smoke, it was easier not to.

I went to college for a year and didn't smoke. After that year, I dropped out of school because I got a high draft lottery number. I decided that I was going to seek my fame and fortune and set off on a little odyssey. I was going to go to Mexico but Paul, a friend of mine, was living in Phoenix. I stopped by to see him and ended up staying. I hung out with him and his friends and they smoked. We used to sit in a pancake restaurant and we'd pool our money for an endless pot of coffee. We'd drink coffee all night with lots of cream and sugar and smoke cigarettes. We had a little "group leader" who was quite a bit older than the rest of us and he set the tone. We drank our coffee the way he liked it. I really started smoking because of peer pressure. They weren't trying to get me to smoke but I wanted to be like them so I smoked. It seemed really cool.

I had experimented a little bit with smoking when I was much younger. I remember once

picking some weeds that were called Indian tobacco. I tried smoking them and scorched my
lungs. For a couple of days in the ninth grade, I
briefly hung out with some guys who smoked
and I remember stealing some cigarettes from my
grandmother and smoking them. I got sick trying
to be cool and I couldn't imagine ever smoking
for real.

Smoking for real in Phoenix wasn't easy at
first. Even drinking the coffee was hard. I had to
put lots of cream and sugar in it to weaken it;
and then to smoke cigarettes, I really had to work
at it. As I recall, my friends mildly discouraged
me because it was so hard for me. Our brand was
Benson & Hedges, the sophisticated brand at the
time, which was kind of a joke because we were
consciously trying not to be sophisticated. It
probably took me a good month or so before I really could smoke a pack a day. But then I got addicted.

By smoking I felt a sense of belonging and very
soon, of course, smoking became a good old
friend. When I'd light one up, I'd feel better. It
was both social and ceremonial. We had these really intense discussions about human needs while
drinking coffee and puffing up a storm at the
pancake house. I have good associations with
smoking at that time.

After smoking for about a year, I felt like I
should quit. I was living in Chicago at the time.
One day I was playing Frisbee in a parking lot
and I was so winded I couldn't believe it. It was
such a foreign experience to feel so winded. I

figured I needed to quit smoking. One day shortly thereafter, I did throw away my pack until I retrieved it about five in the afternoon. I tried to quit a couple times while living in Chicago, but it never went anywhere. I stopped smoking Benson & Hedges and switched to Old Golds before moving back home, where I returned to school in January 1974.

I was living with friends and I remember vividly when Tom, Dick, and I were going to quit smoking. We were going to the university. At the time, I had a part-time job as a Xerox machine operator. One Sunday night we swore off cigarettes and on Monday we all went off to class with no cigarettes. I made it a whole week and it was really hard. On Friday night we were going to a party after I got done working. I went into my boss's office to turn in my time card and there was a pack of cigarettes on her desk. Nobody would know. I looked around and held the cigarette, rolling it in my hands, and I said, "Nope! I quit. I'm not having it." I was so proud of myself. I went to the party and Tom and Dick were smoking. Dick had snuck a cigarette on Tuesday and I felt so betrayed. I lit up a cigarette and I was smoking a pack a day within a day or two.

I didn't think smoking was a good thing to be doing but I didn't think it was all that bad a thing to be doing either. I knew that there were health risks associated with it but I minimized them or joked about it. Several of the people I hung out with smoked so it was really a social thing.

About a year after that, I met Mary (who is

now my wife). When she went into treatment for chemical dependency, I felt like I should quit something too. So I quit cigarettes. It was sort of a noble cause. That was the only reason I was even trying to quit. I would not have been motivated to try and quit otherwise. It was physically difficult to quit; psychologically and emotionally I was very upset because her counselor wouldn't let me see or talk to her. After Mary had been in treatment a couple weeks, I went with my friend, Marty, and his girlfriend from Chicago, to the Boundary Waters of Minnesota. I was still in withdrawal from the nicotine and I was emotionally messed up about Mary being in treatment. I didn't know what was happening. I really missed the cigarettes because I had used them for killing emotional pain and I had a lot of emotional pain in those years.

I remember telling myself that I can't really quit if I'm quitting for someone else or with someone else. Thinking back to when I quit with Dick and Tom, I really wasn't motivated. I felt more like I was quitting for me when Mary was in treatment and I stayed off cigarettes for a couple of years that time, even though Mary still smoked.

At times it was difficult being around a smoker. Some of the worst times were at parties. If I had anything to drink, I instantly wanted a cigarette. I remember a guy telling me there was actually some kind of chemical association between the two. It felt like that for me, but I didn't give in. I felt that if Mary could not drink, then I could not smoke.

I started smoking again almost three years later. I had broken up with Mary in the fall of '77 and we'd gone our separate ways. I had finished college and gone to a quarter of graduate school before I dropped out. I was very heavily involved with some other men in meditation training. I was working and doing the meditation. These friends smoked quite heavily although I had not started yet. We did a training that was twelve weeks long that first spring. It was pretty intense, and I did a couple of meditation programs that winter. Throughout training there was no smoking and no caffeine allowed during the week, although we could drink caffeine on the weekends. We had a particular diet to follow, too, except nobody did. These guys had to quit smoking. It was an intense experience and we had a little closing ceremony at the end of twelve weeks. It was a sense of accomplishment because we had abstained from a variety of things. Finishing the training was worth celebrating. The guys were thrilled because they could have a cigarette, although nobody smoked that first night. Then, the next day, we all smoked, even me. I really got into it again, and for quite awhile I smoked.

I quit again for a brief time when I got sick. I did that several times. Whenever I was sick, I didn't want to smoke. I'd go three, four, or five days without smoking but then start again. The next major time I quit was with Mary. We had gotten back together and married. We had joined a health club in order to clean up our act. We quit smoking and began to work out. It was really hard, really painful. Physically and psychologically the withdrawal was really intense. I had an incredible craving for nicotine. It was like a third hand reaching out of my chest for a cigarette. I got through the craving using intense overexercise. I started swimming and chewed a lot of gum and used sheer force of will. The exercise was helpful, and I ate sugar.

After being off cigarettes for three or four months, we went on a trip. Mary hadn't lasted as long as me. After about two months she had started smoking again which made it very hard for me. I really felt betrayed and it was annoying to be around her when she was smoking.

It still wasn't easy for me to not smoke but I was doing okay. We went on our trip in this little bitty car with Mary puffing away. It was an extremely stressful situation. We'd been to my stepbrother's wedding, and we were heading east. We drove for an hour and a half and realized we'd forgotten our cassette tapes for the trip so we drove back to get them. We lost three hours and we ran into an incredible rainstorm. Before long I was pumping adrenaline and was totally stressed out. Mary was smoking and finally, when the weather broke a little, I lit a cigarette. So we had smoking in common. It was like a social lubricant. Smoking with a friend, at a very physical level, was establishing a meaningful connection, a real bond. By this time, Mary and I were having lots of difficulties in our relationship, and smoking was one of the few things that we could share.

I got really rolling on smoking again on that trip which was the fall of '82. I continued smoking heavily until the next spring. I kept saying I should quit, but I didn't. Not until I got a call from my mom one night. I was home alone, sitting at my desk, smoking cigarettes. She said that my dad was in the hospital and he had cancer. The surgery was already scheduled. I took the cigarette out of my mouth and put it out. That was my last cigarette. Smoking was not fun anymore. I really had a different motivation this time. I knew smoking was threatening. It really hit home that smoking could kill me. I was through kidding myself.

The next two days were just awful, but then it was over pretty much. In many respects, it was the easiest time I ever quit. The first morning my nerve ends were just screaming from the withdrawal; because of my dad, I was not in a good place anyway. I was freaked out. I'd always used cigarettes to suppress my emotions, and facing this with my dad with no painkiller was horrible. It was just awful to feel. Everything was too loud, and too close. I lived through two days of hell. And then it seemed to pass. For that I was grateful. It was much less difficult than all the other times. My Higher Power was able to make it easier for me. I couldn't handle much of anything at the time.

It's about three and a half years now since I've smoked. I've learned that trying to quit for someone else is a lot harder. Knowing the health risks because of my dad's experience gave me motivation that I didn't have the other times I quit.

The benefits of not smoking are great. I'm no longer destroying my clothes and my furniture on a regular basis. My wife and I had spent $2,500 on a real nice sofa that has been irreparably damaged by our smoking. I no longer burn my fingers on a regular basis, trying to draw the cigarette out of my mouth. I'm not an uncoordinated person but I used to pull the core out between my index and middle fingers and burn myself. I feel a lot better physically. I'm exercising regularly and I'm in much better shape than I ever believed possible. Even if I don't exercise at all, I'm still in much better shape. I don't have chronic colds all winter long. I think I probably did permanent damage to my nose from smoking, although I don't have sinus problems anymore. One of the benefits of quitting is that even if you have damaged all those nerves and membranes in your nose, you still can taste things a lot better. I like the way things smell. Our house and my new car smell so good. There are no burns in the upholstery.

I'm pretty confident I'll never smoke again although I don't think I would bet my life on it. If the people really close to me started again, it would make it harder for me. But I have a realization that I hadn't had before about how harmful smoking is.

I'm a happy nonsmoker. I like not smoking. I don't miss it; when I see other people smoke, I'm glad it's not me. I'm free, I hope forever.

MARJORIE

Age 57. Divorced mother of four who is also a recovering alcoholic; loves people, plants, and horses, and is active in community affairs.

The first time I smoked was when I was fifteen. I was with a friend whom I rode horses with. In fact, we were working with our horses that first time I smoked. A lot of people I knew smoked. My mother smoked and all of my friends were beginning to smoke too. I smoked most of my high school years until I was a senior. At that time, I wanted a new horse, one in particular very badly, so I made a deal with my father. If he'd buy me the horse, I wouldn't smoke until I was 21, and I would get on the "A" honor roll. I would have sold my soul for that particular animal. I quit without any difficulty and didn't start again for a while although I smoked before reaching 21.

I started again in college, my freshman year. Most of my friends smoked. I preferred to smoke. It was a good companion. I was not very socially adept; on a date or at a party, smoking gave me something to do, particularly if I was at a loss for words. For nearly 40 years I smoked.

When I hit my forties, I began to notice I was getting short of breath and I knew it was from the smoking. I was leading an extremely active outdoor life by then and whenever I had to run, I was in trouble. My husband and I had bought a farm and I ended up with a boarding stable, our

151

own horses, plus I was taking in boarders. I ended up giving riding lessons. I hadn't intended for this business to get that big. The horse business is like that. It was a busy time for me. I was working in the barn and riding every day and on my feet teaching lessons. Aside from my smoking and drinking, I was physically very fit. The shortness of breath from the smoking was not bad enough to consider quitting. Besides, I had a lot of denial. Other people would get emphysema and lung cancer but I wouldn't.

In these last ten or twelve years of my life, many things have changed that I hadn't counted on. For one, I quit drinking. I got divorced. I changed my vocation; I trained as a chemical dependency counselor and worked at that for a while. But I decided that wasn't what I wanted to do. Through all of this I had a lot of emotional pain, and I kept on smoking. In A.A. there was always support for smoking. Only very, very recently, within the last couple of years, has there been enough awareness to favor nonsmoking A.A. groups.

I began to realize in the last five years that my physical stamina wasn't what I wanted it to be. It was deteriorating. Living in a two-story house, going up and down stairs, was getting harder all the time. I was averaging about a pack-and-a-half a day and I had been doing it for a long time. One of the reasons that I had never tried to stop, even when I was experiencing consequences, was because I was positive I couldn't, and it was not a piece of information I wanted to find out about myself. I felt doomed to keep on smoking. I was not taking part in physical activities because I knew that it would be too hard for me. About six years ago, I tried to play racquetball with a friend. I almost died. I decided not to do *that* again. And that's why I don't play tennis anymore. At the present time, I'm trying to force myself to take walks, but I've never liked walking. I always thought walking was an extraordinarily boring way to spend time. So much has changed since I no longer have the horses. I'm not living that terribly active outdoor life anymore. Everything about my physical life and circumstances has changed.

Before I stopped, many of my friends began talking to me about quitting smoking. I was very cool about it but I felt very defensive inside. I realized my breathing sounded bad, and that was embarrassing. That was another reason I would not exert myself in certain ways when I was around people. I didn't want them to notice. Eventually I realized that unless I did something about my smoking I was going to need one of those cute little portable respirators for sure. I just knew it. I wasn't afraid of cancer. Somehow or other cancer was not a concern of mine. I wasn't afraid of dying of lung cancer but I was afraid of living with a little oxygen tube in my nose. They don't look very cute.

I kept putting quitting off, but I was beginning to say to myself, every time I lit a cigarette, this is it. The internal dialogue was beginning to take place, but it took two years of self-talk to quit. I sort of tiptoed around it, looking over my shoulder every now and then. I'd look but I wasn't able to face the issue squarely.

Finally, I tried a couple of things to help me quit. On a whim one day, I bought antismoking stuff at the drugstore that you chew. It was not Nicorette gum. These were tablets that made your cigarettes taste absolutely awful. I brought the tablets home, stuck them in the back of my closet, and left them there. Six months or a year later, I dug them out and thought, oh, gee, maybe I'll try this. At first I was able to cut down on my smoking but, just like controlled drinking, it was too hard. At first, though, I was very encouraged by that and thought, well, at least I know that I can smoke less. It was a very slow process for me. But I found that I couldn't keep it up. It was just too hard. And so I let the whole thing go for a while and returned to smoking just like before.

Next I talked with somebody about acupuncture. And probably six months after that, I got acupuncture. At the same time I also got a Nicorette gum prescription from my doctor. I'd also gotten some information about a Twelve Step program for not smoking. Using the Twelve Step program didn't work at all for me. Although I'd never liked gum, chewing the Nicorettes was helpful somewhat during the physical withdrawal. And the acupuncture helped at first. But the effect wasn't long-lasting. I think all the acupuncture did was mask the withdrawal symptoms. However, by using all these tools, I managed not to smoke for about a week, which was an improvement. But again it was just too hard not to smoke. It was just too hard. So I ended up going back to it. I started by thinking, oh, I'll just have one. I can't remember how long it took me to get back up to my pack-and-a-half a day, but not long enough.

A short time later I was at a meeting, and a woman about my age announced that she hadn't smoked for a full year. I hadn't known her very well, but I sort of raised my ears. I wanted to know what she did — what worked for her. So I asked her about it. She had gone through a program called Clean Break. She had tried acupuncture and many other things unsuccessfully. Finally, Clean Break had worked for her. Shortly thereafter, I saw their ad in the newspaper. The ad said if you're interested in quitting, just bring your cigarettes and an open mind. That's what I did. In many ways it's a hard-line program. And in some ways it's like A.A. because it's taught by ex-smokers — not doctors. The guy who ran the section I went to said, "You're all a bunch of junkies." You could just feel the tension in the room.

They talked a lot about deprivation. Deprivation is what makes people return to smoking. They gave us some tools to help us deal with that. One of the tools was telephone counseling. We could call a group leader anytime for support. And the leader called me twice a week. He said that one of the reasons people fail when they try to stop smoking is they immediately want to call themselves nonsmokers. He didn't believe it was possible for a smoker to ever really feel like a nonsmoker. He said, "It's a little bit like turning back into a cucumber after you're pickled." Not everyone will agree with all parts of this program, but it helped me. However, I've never been so sick in my life as since I stopped smoking.

It has been about a year-and-a-half since I smoked, and I've never felt so bereft in my life. Smoking was like my lover and I feel abandoned. The reason I quit when I did was because I was planning a trip to Canada. I knew I would be hiking a lot and I wanted not to be so short of breath. On the trip I felt fine. I walked all over the place and I wasn't breathless. I had also planned a trip to England following the Canadian trip. But when I landed in the airport, I couldn't breathe. I could barely make it from the airplane through the airport to the bus that was going to take us where my friend and I were going. Although the doctors in England couldn't find anything wrong with me, I could barely get out of bed. I ended up coming home early. I felt like I was living in a dead body. I was scared. I was literally only able to do the bare minimum necessary for survival. I went to my doctor and he couldn't find a thing wrong with me either. That was even more disturbing.

Finally a friend took me to a chiropractor and holistic healer. She gave me Adrenalin and diagnosed a number of problems that made perfect sense to me. She said that my entire system had gotten so dependent on the stimulation from nicotine that it had just quit working without it.

I'm still in the process of getting back to normal. I'm doing very little. I had started a business with a friend but I had to drop out. I just couldn't keep it up. Emotionally, I was a mess. I've come to the conclusion that I used cigarettes to cope so extensively that it was like losing the Band-Aid. I had no idea how important nicotine was in my life. Without it, I cried inappropriately. The only reason I haven't gone back to smoking is that I want to live more than I want to die. And I never want to go through quitting again. I'd rather sober up every other week from alcohol than go through what I have the past year-and-a-half. It has been the hardest time I've ever put in. Ever! I couldn't have made it without friends I could just babble to. And babble I did. It did not occur to me to go to a Smokers Anonymous group. I didn't have the energy.

Although not smoking has been very hard, there are some pluses; the best thing about not smoking is being free of the control it had over me. I like not having to run back and get my cigarettes or make sure I have them whenever I go out. I'm not feeling all that much better physically than before I stopped, but I am breathing a little better. I've put on more weight than I wanted to, but I was terribly underweight when I quit smoking so that's probably not all bad.

Also I'm not fighting with myself all the time now that I've quit. I had reached the point where I was feeling guilty every time I lit a cigarette. And that was not fun. I'm free now of the preoccupation with cigarettes. But the most important thing someone needs in order to successfully quit is a good support group. It took me several attempts to quit smoking; however, I'm glad I kept trying.

Recently I've realized that how I think about myself has changed a lot since I quit. The change is the result of not smoking, but it's not just the not smoking. I'm more concerned these days with getting physically healed and getting some energy back. I've gotten into more psychological and emotional growth too. Stopping smoking for me has triggered a whole new phase of living. My feelings are no longer muffled. Smoking was how I coped with emotional things, with issues of all kinds. The Band-Aid has been removed, but the owie's still there. Sometimes it's threatening. Sometimes it's infuriating because growth is terribly, terribly slow. There are times when I would much prefer to be back where I was as a smoker, but it would be really stupid to start smoking again and I don't like thinking of myself as stupid.

I remember going to work right after I quit and being absolutely good for nothing at all. I literally did not know what I was doing or where I was going. I had to be led around by my hand which, in a sense, can be very reinforcing. I did find out that my friends loved me no less as a blithering idiot. That was strengthening. I think smoking is an addiction for most of us. There aren't many people like my mother who tapered off. It's for certain I couldn't do it like that.

Quitting is the hardest thing I've ever done and I have no explanation for it. I used smoking as a substitute for everything and I'm still in the process of grieving and it's been a year-and-a-half. It's almost as if the deprivation of the cigarettes was like a magnet and everything in my life that I'd never grieved was drawn to the surface. This has been a very difficult period for me. I find I need a lot of reassurance that this too shall pass. But I'm hopeful. And I'm glad I'm no longer smoking. I've learned it is possible to live without smoking, and I was not sure of that a little more than eighteen months ago.

JOHN

*Age 28. Engineer; married, and a
new father; talented trumpet player;
woodworking hobbiest, and home re-
modeler.*

I started smoking on a work crew with a
bunch of kids my age. We were digging trenches
for phone lines. I was about fifteen and I wanted
to feel as though I belonged. One of the group
had a pack of cigarettes so we all smoked. Prior
to that, the kids I hung out with didn't smoke.
Peer pressure had a lot to do with my starting.

I remember the very first time. It was powerful stuff. It made me dizzy and my heart
pounded. The rush of the drug really got me. It
wasn't really pleasurable. Actually I felt nauseous
but in order to maintain my "in" with the group,
I kept doing it. And then the effects became less.
From age fifteen on I was a regular smoker and I
smoked a pack a day.

While growing up, before I started smoking, I
more or less expected to smoke eventually (because many of my older brothers did) even
though I was into athletics a bit. Many of my
older sisters smoked too. My mother never
smoked and my father only smoked a pipe for a
while when I was very, very young. I don't think
he ever smoked cigarettes.

By the time I was sixteen, I had reduced my
athletics to skiing. I was on the ski team but I
didn't compete. I just went out to ski. There were
rules about not smoking so I would hide out with

it. I also played in the school band and it was not acceptable to smoke there but we hid it. Because my mother had fallen on her head years before, she had lost her sense of smell; thus, I was able to smoke at home and get away with it. She didn't approve of my smoking but she couldn't tell when I was doing it.

In fact, my friends and I smoked pot and cigarettes in the basement. It was okay with my father if our friends smoked cigarettes in the house. That was acceptable. We couldn't, but it was okay if they did. If someone lit a cigarette, then it didn't matter whether it was pot smoke or something else in the air. My friends smoking was also a means of covering up the whole pot smoking situation.

I really enjoyed smoking from the very first, but it became such an obsession. Early on, smoking ran me rather than my running it, so I did quit on more than one occasion for brief spells.

I was nineteen and a college student the first time I quit. I realized every time a tense situation came up, I reached for the cigarettes. The lie about smoking was that it was going to get me through the situation and I'd feel better. Smoking was going to handle the situation for me. That was the big lie although I definitely believed it at the time.

I was a musician while in school. I played the trumpet in the band and smoking affected my wind. It had become such an obsession by this time. I had already quit drinking and suddenly I had an increased awareness about what was going on with my body. I was playing my horn a lot and smoking was affecting my lung power, so I decided to quit. In preparation, I worked with a guy who did hypnosis with me. He was a university psychologist who worked in human development. He taught me self-hypnosis using visualization and meditation. He taught me techniques of relaxation to combine with the self-hypnosis. I saw him on a weekly basis for a couple of months while I was tapering down on my smoking. Eventually, I had some luck with abstaining.

The sessions were structured in three parts. We did visualization and meditation. In the meditation, I'd sit down, close my eyes, and take a deep breath to relax. Then I'd concentrate on three main principles. One was that smoking was poison for my body. The second one was I needed my body to live. The third principle was that I owed myself the respect of protection and consideration. He instructed me to also do some association with pleasurable things that I would get out of not smoking. For instance, being able to have the lung power to blow my horn, to be really "hot" on the horn; another was the ability to enjoy the taste of food again; also just getting rid of the messy habit of smoking. He helped me to remember pleasurable experiences from my past when I was a nonsmoker. He'd suggest I visualize myself in a favorite place in the world. And then he'd bring me back to the three principles and thereby formed an association between the two. The technique worked for me. Shortly thereafter,

I transferred to another university as a non-smoker.

Unfortunately, it wasn't long lasting. By springtime, I started smoking again. The day I started was a tough day. My car had failed to start and I had to hitchhike to school. Who should come along but some of my old friends from high school, whom I hadn't seen in quite some time. They picked me up and they were all smoking. For some time I had failed to do the daily three point visualization and meditation the hypnotist had taught me. And I started smoking again. It was just like the first time I ever smoked. I got the good rush. But that time I didn't feel nauseous and dizzy with the pounding heart. None of the negative consequences were there. It felt good to smoke. After all, I was having a tough day and I thought, why not? Smoking felt friendly and familiar.

I smoked for another four years then but it wasn't long before it was not very satisfying. Once again, I had the delusion that it somehow made problems easier to handle. By the time I got around to working on quitting again, I was out of school and working as an engineer, trying to be professional. Oftentimes people would call with difficult situations and I'd find myself reaching for the pack of cigarettes. Again, I was haunted by the same lie, believing that smoking would somehow get me through the difficult situations. For me, one of the keys of successfully quitting was that I had to quit lying to myself about what cigarettes did and did not do for me.

Eventually, I reached a point of being fed up with the habit and how it had me. I didn't have it. I realized that it was a lie. Smoking never did help me through any situation. Talking with other people who were also struggling to quit was real helpful. On my 24th birthday I quit for the last time and that was four years ago on November 20th.

I didn't choose to quit on my birthday for any special reason. I'd been hoping to quit for a long time, but I still was walking around with cigarettes. On that day I'd left them in the car and was moving from one place to the other in a friend's vehicle without my cigarettes. That was the first night I went without. It was tough. I had strong cravings but as long as I kept myself occupied it was a little easier. The desire to smoke was mostly mental, but I think the mental is triggered by the physical reaction. I had been smoking a pack a day and it had been consistent day after day.

After quitting, I began to involve myself with groups that didn't smoke. I sought out people who were either not smoking or who were sharing the struggle to not smoke. I soon learned that no urge ever lasts more than 30 seconds. I could deal with each little urge and get through that. I recalled that the first thing that happens when you take a drag off a cigarette is that you get a big breath of air as well. So I started just taking deep breaths. There's something relaxing and satisfying just taking a big breath now. I was gentle with myself the day I finally quit. Finally quitting was the culmination of quite a period of working up to it.

Another tool that I learned when I'd quit an earlier time was when I found myself reaching for a cigarette, I'd draw my hand back and gently rub my cheek. I was changing my behavior and being nice to myself. It's the same movement to bring a cigarette up to your lips as bringing your hand up to your cheek, but the gentle touch to the cheek is like giving yourself a gift.

Even though I haven't smoked now for four years, there have been a couple times, while getting together with people who were enjoying their cigarettes, that I really wanted one. But generally they look bad. They smell bad. I don't like to be around anyone who is smoking. I don't like them to be around me. I don't like for people to smoke in the house, my car, or my workstation. I sit in an area at work that's no smoking. When people bring cigarettes over unconsciously, I ask them not to smoke in my area. More and more, the people I associate with don't smoke. I think that people who have quit are moving toward higher spiritual things and cleaning up their act entirely.

I had only smoked for eight years which isn't long but it affected my lung capacity. It affected me to a great extent. I thought smoking made me attractive but that's hardly true. It turned away people that I might have met otherwise. I shun smokers now. I don't like to be around them because it offends me, so I'm sure others stayed away from me. I probably missed meeting some marvelous people.

There are so many rewards for not smoking but the best reward is I'm not polluting the air. Also, my baby will grow up with a role model who doesn't smoke. That's important to me. I'm finding healthier ways to relax and more positive ways to deal with the trials of life. I relax through deep breathing, along with using meditation and visualization. It really helps. It really calms me down. Not smoking is a conscious choice. Smoking was not a conscious choice. It was beyond choosing. It was automatic.

Whenever I feel I'm wavering, I remember the three point meditation: Smoking is poison for my body. I need my body to live. I owe myself that respect. And then I visualize being able to taste my food, breathing deeply, and smelling good. The urges won't last more than 30 seconds. I don't beat myself up if I long for a cigarette. Any addiction is powerful stuff. My first cigarette just about knocked me over. In my mind, it's as hard as any other drug to give up, and it doesn't get you through tough situations. It doesn't make anything any easier. Smoking isn't handsome or beautiful or sophisticated. It's a lie to believe otherwise.

It's pretty rare now that I get an urge to smoke again, and I'm very happy not smoking. I'm really happy living in a house that doesn't smell like smoke. It feels safe knowing that we won't cause a fire from careless smoking. It's nice to be alive. I get good feelings knowing that I'm free, that smoking isn't controlling me. My father died of cancer, not from smoking, but that had a profound effect on me because smoking is so associated with cancer. I watched the slow disintegration of a very big man to a very small person. The cancer just ate him up. I feel good being alive and I guess that's the key for me. I like being alive and I don't want to contribute in any way to an untimely, early death! Not smoking is a good choice for me.

TERENCE

*Age 50. An attorney; married and the
father of four; loves escaping to his
condo in Snowmass, Colorado, to ski.*

I don't remember the first cigarette that I ever
had, although I was about fifteen, and I smoked
because everybody else was having a cigarette.
Nobody in my family smoked, but all my friends
did. We smoked Luckies or Chesterfields, and I
became an avid smoker from the very start. It
was a big thing to have a whole carton of Luckies
or Chesterfields. Even though I started smoking
with my friends, I smoked at home right away.
Nobody objected. When I think back about it, I
didn't particularly enjoy smoking. I smoked because everybody else did. It never did anything
special for me but I smoked anyway.

Most of the places I went prohibited smoking
— at school, for example. But we smoked anyway and occasionally got caught. We'd have a
cigarette before we went into school. Generally
we'd go somewhere out on the football field, far
away from detection.

While in high school I had a job in a drugstore. I noted very soon the only way I could get
a break was to have a cigarette and a cup of coffee. I think I started smoking cigarettes and
drinking coffee at the same time so that I could
take a break. It was the one sure way to get one. I
continued smoking when I went off to college.
During this early period of my life, I never considered not smoking. I smoked all through college

and law school. I smoked continually until I was about 30. Smoking had begun to feel like a good friend. Even now I can practically feel the cigarette between my fingers. If I take a deep breath, I get some satisfaction from the experience.

While I was in high school, most of my friends smoked, but in college very few did. In law school there were even fewer people my age who smoked. Because of that, I experimented with stopping many times. I was not able to stop smoking for good the first time I tried.

As I recall, my first experience with trying to quit was prior to starting law school. I thought it would be good discipline for me not to smoke in law school. I'd be much smarter and much better in school, I thought. There must have been something detrimental about smoking in my mind although I don't recall the specifics any longer. But after a very short time I started smoking again. I wasn't able to go more than a day or two without a cigarette. I do remember though that even for that day or two, I felt better.

The next time I remember quitting was four or more years later after I was married and living in Washington. I had finished law school. The Surgeon General had made his first report about the dangers of smoking. That was in 1963 or so. My wife quit smoking at that time, and she pressured me to quit. Once again, I did for a brief period, this time a week or so. Soon thereafter, I started smoking again but not at home. I smoked outside of the house on the sly. My wife could probably smell it on me. So she probably knew long before

I admitted I was smoking. By this time, smoking was not consistent with my values, but I did it anyway.

I kept starting and stopping in those days, at least two or three more times. I had stopped once; I was in New York and it was very cold. I was very miserable, so I started smoking again. Another time I remember starting again during a long automobile trip. I was moving back to my home state from Washington. I passed a drugstore advertising cigarettes for $1.90 a carton which was very inexpensive, so I got a carton for the trip home. I was traveling alone and I proceeded to smoke all the way home. My wife had gone by plane. I was disappointed and felt guilty that I started again. I figured by this time that I wasn't able to quit. I felt that smoking was one of the few things that I wasn't able to control at that point in my life. I think that's why I kept trying to stop. But finally I was successful.

I was very sick at the time. I had the flu and could barely lift my head off the pillow and I was still looking for a cigarette. But it tasted just awful and made me more sick. I finally concluded that if it tasted that bad and I could be that sick and still want one, it was time to quit. Quitting this time was a little easier because I was so sick the first few days that I was off. I had been smoking for twenty years.

For the first few weeks after quitting my concentration wasn't good. My job requires heavy concentration and part of the regime of concentration was to have a cigarette. Without that, I searched for a lot of substitutes. For a while I used a pencil routine. I held the pencil between my fingers like a cigarette. It took a month or two before the really intense desire to smoke died down. It was another six months or more until the smell of a cigarette didn't make me want one. Often if I had a drink, I'd want a cigarette. Since my pattern had been to have a cigarette after dinner, I began to eat chocolate sundaes as a substitute. Fortunately, I didn't gain weight. I was eating other sugary treats during the day, too, as a substitute. Unlike some people, I didn't get into physical activity. I'm a skier now but it wasn't something I took up to replace smoking. I didn't necessarily get into healthier things as a result of not smoking. I considered not smoking enough all by itself.

I don't miss smoking anymore, but it took quite awhile to get to that point. I did have a cigarette once in the early seventies. It was a victory celebration after an election and everybody was having one. It tasted very good, but my wife and my friends quickly got on my case about it. I think if I had had a second one, I would be smoking today. It's possible to go back and I don't want to. I would be right back to where I was before all too quickly, smoking a pack a day in no time.

The best reward of not smoking is that I don't feel tied to cigarettes. I became dependent on them very quickly and they became a part of everything that I did. While I was smoking, I couldn't enjoy things without having a cigarette.

One of the most difficult things about not smoking was that all of the parts of my life had been invaded by cigarettes. Now, though, I feel good about the real freedom to enjoy things without cigarettes.

My experience taught me that if you really want to quit, just keep trying. Even though I was not successful the first or the second or the third time, each time I tried, I learned a little more about myself and what it took to quit. For every smoker who wants to quit, at some point, the right circumstances will come along and make it possible to stick with quitting. Getting support from others helps. Although, at the time I quit, I didn't understand the value of support. My idea was that quitting was a matter of character. If I decided on a course of action, then I had to follow through. I was supposed to overcome whatever my problem was. That I failed to stay with quitting really bothered me.

Not many people smoked when I quit, so I didn't have friends who could offer support. If I were quitting today, I'd sign up for a stop-smoking program and get the support that would make it easier. But I'm glad that my experience of quitting is now behind me.

JAMES

*Age 75. Retired real estate developer
and tax accountant; father of eight,
married 48 years; enjoys gardening
and civic affairs.*

I started smoking when I was about fifteen.
My brother, Leo, who was two years older, had
already started. Originally, we always smoked together. Unfortunately, he never was able to quit
even when he needed to. He died of lung cancer
when he was 46. He had willpower, strength,
and character, but he could not quit smoking.
And he tried a thousand times. Leo and I used to
have bets on quitting smoking at Lent. I could always quit for Lent, but he couldn't. I smoked
from age fifteen on for better than 50 years, but I
quit a lot of times between 1926 and 1979.

Growing up, most of the boys I knew smoked
with the exception of a couple of my older brothers. Smoking had only become popular about ten
years earlier. The thing I liked about smoking
from the very first was the sedative feeling it gave
me. It calmed me down a little bit. Another
thing I liked was being like everyone else. It was
the thing to do. While in high school, we always
smoked in the "john" at recess. I imagine 75 percent of the boys smoked. Just twenty years earlier, around 1915, nobody smoked.

One of the reasons it became quickly popular
was that it was cheap. Cigarettes were twelve to
fifteen cents a pack; only ten cents for certain
ones. There were Lucky Strikes, Chesterfields,

and Camels. There was one kind in a purple or a light blue package but I can't remember the brand. They were all small cigarettes. There were no filters and no king-size cigarettes back then. I think there was a little more tobacco in them then and fewer chemicals, but they were still as habit-forming. They were very, very tough to quit.

I started trying to quit smoking when I was only twenty. I was working my first real job, and I spent ten bucks out of my first paycheck and sent away for a "how to quit smoking kit" that I saw advertised in a magazine. The program did not work. I wanted to quit because I didn't like to be controlled by cigarettes. I was not in control and I wanted to quit permanently but I just couldn't. I was able to quit for Lent for 20 or 30 different years, so I knew I could do it, but I'd always go back. One time I quit for a year. Back then I used to frequently go on the wagon. I had been a drinker all my life and when I'd quit drinking periodically, I'd notice that my need for cigarettes was greater. When I was doing my normal drinking, it was much simpler not to smoke.

I came to really know smoking as a terrible habit and a serious health hazard, in time. When I finally had my lung operation, I was about 68. Nobody told me I had to quit when the operation was over, but I did, even though I didn't end up having lung cancer. I had two spots on my lungs that weren't cancer. Surprisingly, I didn't have any negative side effects from my smoking or my drinking for many years. Apparently, I had an unusual cast-iron stomach and constitution. However, the operation on my lungs, even though the spots were benign, proved to be terrible. They had to break my ribs and everything. It took me four or five months to get over it. That ended up being the major negative side effect until some years later. Due to the operation, I lost at least a third of my respiratory velocity. My shortness of breath is the result.

My surgery for throat cancer this past summer affected my breathing capacity even more. A couple of doctors told me that these operations were similar to open-heart surgery. They figure a 10 to 15 percent loss of lung capacity because they have to break the bronchial tubes and when they put them back together, they never have that same elasticity. In my case, I think that I had probably 85 or 90 percent capacity before the first lung operation because my doctor, several years before, had tested me out on some steps in his office, and my lungs were strong.

Before cancer surgery this past summer, my capacity was at 67 percent. Now I'm down to less than 30 percent. I'm certain that this last operation on my throat was directly caused by my smoking even though I quit seven years ago and quitting was not as hard as I had expected because I didn't feel I had a choice. I felt that if I didn't quit I probably would have died, particularly with the reduced lung capacity. It makes it a little easier to quit when the odds are against you. I quit because I was forced to if I wanted to live.

Within just a few months after I quit, my senses of smell and taste showed a tremendous difference. It seemed my sense of smell got sharper all the time. It was especially nice when we were out in the country. There were some pretty nice smells out there in the spring and I noticed them. My sense of taste was sharpened considerably and I gained some weight but that was okay because I was recovering from the operation which had affected my appetite. But after that, I had to watch my weight a little more than before.

Even though quitting was easier than I had anticipated, I did crave cigarettes but it seemed like each day it was a little better. After about a week, I noticed it was easier, day by day. Then every day for months I used the "one day at a time" game plan. And it worked real well because the desire to smoke continued to be pronounced. I think the desire to smoke is a little different than the desire to take a drink. In the case of smoking, the desire is more pronounced because the temptation to have a cigarette is more frequent than the desire to have a drink. The desire to have a drink comes at a party or while going past a bar, but the smoking desire is constant. Taking it one day at a time was a great help to me.

The thing that led up to my last operation was just a bad cold that I couldn't shake and a sore throat that wasn't really very sore. However, I should have taken action faster than I did. And, of course, I can't help but blame my family doctor because I went to him in February with this cold and each time I told him my throat was sore, he'd tell me to take cough medicine. In May, the throat was still sore and I'd get coughing spells, usually in the evening. That lasted for over a month while I still had this slight soreness. I criticize myself severely now for not having gone to another doctor sooner.

On the fifteenth of May, I went to an ear, nose, and throat specialist. I told him about my sore throat and he said it was a little viral infection. Then on the fifth of June, I finally went back to my family doctor and I screamed. I said, "This sore throat is not going away and there's something screwy." He sent me to a specialist. He put a little mirror down my throat and said, "Looks to me like you've got cancer." It was that simple. He said he'd do a biopsy but if he were a betting man, he'd bet on cancer.

I wasn't really surprised. I kind of expected it. As soon as he said, "I can see something down there," I knew. Before then I had never thought of cancer. In my whole lifetime, I've only known two people who had cancer of the throat. And I've known hundreds of them that have had other types of cancer.

I was operated on the third of July and the cancer was pretty far advanced. The first doctor said my whole voice box had to be taken out and the second one said he thought he could save just a little of it, which he did. But I feel that, had I screamed 60 days quicker, it might have turned out differently. I was on the operating table for eight hours. They just had to keep shaving and shaving and shaving on the voice box. I knew my cancer was related to my smoking. I used to think that once you quit you were safe. I don't believe that anymore. I think if you smoke for 50 years like I did, there's a certain amount of permanent damage. Even though it may not cause cancer in everybody, that's a lot of poison in your system, your throat, your lungs, and other parts of your body.

I came from a big family and many people died of cancer. There were twelve children in my family, and I'm the youngest of six boys. Three girls were younger than me but my oldest sisters and brothers were twelve to fourteen years older than I was. They all married into other families of ten or twelve children. My oldest sister got married in 1923. That was a long time ago. With all of the marrying and connections to bigger families, I'm aware of many relatives and near relatives who died of cancer. I would say in the last five years in this family, there have been at least 35 or 40 cancer deaths. All my life, I've been aware of the cancer deaths. My brother, just older than I, died at age 46 with cancer of the lungs. He was a heavy, heavy smoker. He never could quit. He could do anything else but he couldn't quit. Every time friends or relatives got cancer, I visited them often before they died. I had learned about cancer. One of my cousins died of cancer of the larynx, like mine. I had a friend, a business acquaintance about 25 years ago, who died. He had his voice box removed. Of all the cancer victims I knew, though, they are the only ones with cancer like mine.

Even though I'd watched relatives and friends die for years, I wasn't inspired to quit. And, of course, the older I got, the less need there seemed to be to quit. When you're 72, the actuarial tables are a lot different than when you're 21. Your life expectancy takes on a whole different look. The fear of getting cancer when you're over 70 isn't the same as at 50 or 40. Besides, when you get over 70, somewhere in the next twenty years you're going to die anyway.

It's my personal feeling that it's a shame we don't do more educating at the ten-year-old level so that kids never start. My biggest complaint for a long time has been that the Department of Agriculture subsidizes farmers to grow tobacco to kill the American people.

Since my surgery, I've had tremendous difficulty learning how to eat and drink. The eating has been especially hard. It's been 90 days since I had surgery, and I'm still having a lot of difficulty swallowing. I've had to learn to swallow a new way. And, if I'm not careful, I get a tickling that will throw me into a coughing spell that can really be frightening — I'm not too sure that I'm going to be able to stop sometimes. There have been a couple times that have really scared the heck out of me. The swallowing is hard because to remove the malignant cancer cells, they had to interfere with the windpipe, and the windpipe and the pipe that our food goes down are similarly related. We all know what it feels like to get food down our windpipe. This happens a lot after this operation. I have to put my neck way to one side and try to get the food to go down on the opposite side of where the surgery was performed. I don't know how much longer it's going to take to master this.

I still have a semiparalysis, a numbness in my ear and my neck and my tongue, too. It's just the most terrible operation. I hope I'm not going to need radiation because the doctors tell me that there are many nerve cells in your neck and that the first application of radiation kills those nerves. Many of those nerves have to do with the liquefying of a normal amount of mucus that we all develop in our system. The nerves liquefy it and it goes on through our waste system, but when these nerves are killed, the mucus becomes a solid substance and it's an awful problem. The threat of pneumonia is multiplied too.

My voice is gone, even though I can whisper, but my worst problem is my shortness of breath. Even if I had a full voice box, I would still have shortness of breath. But though my problems are many, I am grateful for the pluses in my life. My sense of smell has improved and I feel better knowing that I'm in control of something rather than being controlled. That gives me strength.

For about 25 years at least, the medical evidence has been preponderous. There's absolutely no question that smoking damages one's health. Thirty years ago, 40 years ago, doctors smoked their heads off, but they seldom do anymore. They see the evidence. It's self-evident that smoking is harmful. There isn't any benefit to it; it's tough to get the habit broken, but it can be done.

The money saved from not smoking, particularly at today's prices, is a benefit. I smoked more than two packages a day for years and years and that's a reasonably expensive habit. And it's a dangerous habit. I can think of at least several instances where fires were started and there was no question but that they were caused by cigarettes. Smoking is a dirty habit, and it's nice to own my own soul. Not smoking makes me feel good, I am now in charge instead of letting cigarettes rule me. And with all I've lost as the result of smoking, that's important.

THERESA

Age 37. Married, mother of a one-year-old boy; trained as a nurse and a family therapist; pastime is facilitating mental health in family and friends.

I think what interested me most about smoking, what was most significant, was that it was congruent, that it fit, with my feelings. When I took a drag off the cigarette that I had lit with a match, it burned and made me feel bad. Then I felt congruent. It felt more real than some other things I had experienced around my home. Smoking fit with the experience of discomfort I had around home. I went for the congruency, and for the altered state. I liked the feeling of being out of control.

I started smoking early, at probably eleven or twelve years of age. It was a way to be with friends. It separated me out with people the same way basketball or a writing club or hockey might. We had our smoking club. It was a way that we were together. Probably the least scary way to be in a group was to smoke. We just got together and smoked.

I grew up knowing that smoking was an obvious option for my life. This was probably 1962 and there was no surgeon general's report. It was just another option of being an adult like drinking coffee. It didn't have all the health and moral tags that it has now.

Through high school I smoked off and on because of the availability of time where I could smoke. As soon as it was legal to smoke, when I was eighteen, I was in for a pack-and-a-half a day, and that's where I stayed. It never got more and it never got less. It stayed pretty steady and I never tried to quit. It never crossed my mind to quit for thirteen years. I was quickly into the blindness of the addiction. I can remember standing at six o'clock in the morning, waiting for my ride to nursing school, having had nothing to eat, and smoking. It was 25 degrees below zero and I was smoking on the front porch. I couldn't talk. I was having a fit of coughing and continuing to smoke right through it, just getting enough breath to get my next puff on the cigarette.

As I started to have other things that felt congruent in my life, cigarettes felt less and less so. Telling the truth about who I was, and feeling the sweetness of that; and having someone talk back to me honestly and feeling the joy of that, meant cigarettes filled a need less and less. As those experiences accumulated, then the cloud of denial started to break down. Smoking finally felt less and less compatible with who I was becoming. I was changing. I couldn't smoke in the same way. Finally it no longer fit with how I saw myself.

But the process of quitting took about three years, because of my fear of total withdrawal. I had watched other people quit, and I was living with a nonsmoker. We had certain rules limiting my smoking. I couldn't smoke in the car, and certainly not in the bedroom. My smoking world was getting decreased. I was overcome by the fear of withdrawal and the lack of faith that I could actually live through the terrible withdrawal. I was so aware of physical and psychological discomfort that I tried to quit four or five times, but I wasn't successful. And yet, I could not stand the feeling that came as soon as I started to smoke again.

The first time I quit I tried willpower. I decided I was not going to do it anymore. It was pride. I saw my friends quit, so I did it on sheer willpower. I made it about three or four weeks. And then, in a weak moment, I felt angry, or disgusted or something, and I started again. It was hard to do it by willpower.

Several months later, I went through a behavior modification program. I went to groups. It was a psychological conditioning program. I filled out checks for two dollars each, twenty or more of them. If I broke my commitment to not smoking, I had to send one of the checks to the charity of my choice or whomever I made them out to. I was so determined to quit that I made out the checks to my husband's ex-wife, every single check. The program insisted I send them to her, one at a time with a letter explaining that I had failed in my attempts to quit smoking; therefore, she was going to gain by my failure. I made it for three or four weeks; then I went to the instructor and said, "I can't do this. Sending the checks could be serious family trouble for me." I ended up sending the money to something else.

So, for a second time, I lasted for a few weeks.

Between three and six weeks, I would just crack. It was never the first day. It was the continued pressure of my life-style without smoking. The psychological addiction was pretty much over. The physical addiction was left. My feelings were very much like premenstrual syndrome. I was real irritable, and it felt like I had nerve endings pushing out of my skin. It felt like I was walking through a doorway filled with razor blades and there was just barely enough room for me to get through. I felt like I was getting little tiny cuts all over my entire body. My whole nervous system was a shambles. And again, I went back. It was the six-week mark where it was always hard for me. I went back to smoking at least four times when the worst should have been over.

The next time, I just tried quitting again on my own. My attitude was, okay, now I am going to do it. I started by trying running. I remember reading some place about replacing one addiction with another. I thought, I'll run. Even though I'm smoking, I will start to run. I got out my little shoes and started to run. I ran one block, and I had to walk home. I got up to a mile or a mile-and-a-half and it did cut my smoking down. I didn't smoke for two hours after I ran. But I gave up the running. I was trying all combinations of things to quit. It got pretty ridiculous.

I would smoke Camels without filters. If I wanted to smoke, that was what I got. Pretty soon I got used to them. I was working nights as a nurse. I remember taking Camels, wrapping the whole package in white, surgical tape, real thick, and setting it on the desk. I'd tell the nurse with me, "I'm not going to smoke tonight but I'll just leave these here as an option; it'll take me an hour to get to the cigarettes which will give me time to think about what I'm doing." By three o'clock in the morning I was having an attack, and I cut through the whole package.

At the time, I lived in a real sleazy place where I went to the basement to smoke. I had a chair down there and any time I wanted to smoke, no matter where I was, I had to go to the basement. That cut me down to three cigarettes a day. That helped retrain me for a life-style without cigarettes, but I hung on to those three cigarettes and looked forward to them.

I was suffering consequences in my marriage because of smoking. If I had been smoking and my husband wanted to kiss me, I'd do self-conscious stuff. I was self-conscious about my clothes smelling too. Then about eight or nine years ago, after those two or three years of trying, I quit. This one day, I had been smoking so much that I really felt nauseated, extremely nauseated. I was a student and between classes I'd maybe do ten cigarettes before my next lecture. I thought I was going to throw up and I had a flash, almost like a vision, that I had absolutely no control over the cigarettes. I had this vision of these guys who had control of me, in this little college dorm area. I was in a jail cell with cigarettes, totally locked-up. They had me hand-cuffed. I never picked up a cigarette after that. It was a flood of insight, a paradigm shift. It felt like a spiritual experience. I had some vacation time, and then Christmas vacation came right at my critical six-week mark.

I read a lot of autobiographies. I read about Margaret Mead and Isadora Duncan. Reading about other people's lives helped. One morning I was alone and I saw a cigarette and I lit it. I took one puff. It was so repugnant. It really was as bad as I remembered. It was over. I suddenly realized that I had control over how I felt. That is powerful. And then I got colds. I had respiratory infections for six months. Because of my own struggles, I am empathetic with anyone trying to quit. I feel that smokers are in prison. It is the smelliest habit and I'm glad for my freedom.

There are so many rewards from not smoking. I can remember walking down the street the first spring after quitting and smelling lilacs before I saw them. That was powerful. I didn't know where they were. I looked around and they were a little ways away. That felt like a real gift. Before, I had to have flowers right up to my nose before I could smell them. My sexuality changed too. I no longer had that "I need to brush my teeth" feeling. I also discovered I am a bad cook. I didn't know it before because I couldn't taste the food. I didn't really gain weight, but I did have a shift of metabolism. I didn't have that real scrawny look anymore. I took on about ten pounds but it made me more solid; it wasn't fat.

187

I've never gotten back to that real skinny look.

One thing I had to learn to do was take breaks. I didn't know how to take breaks — especially on Saturday. There was nothing built in. I would go a whole day and never really have sat down and relaxed. The cigarettes always provided me with a natural pause, and I had to train myself to pause.

My smoking days seem so far away. It seems as far away as the girl who was out looking for pot on Friday nights. Bill, my husband, helped me to quit. He didn't enable me to smoke, nor did he hassle me. He never said anything directly to me, but he would say, "Your smoking is bothering me." How could I argue with that? And he wouldn't say, "Would you mind not smoking?" He said, "That is really bothering me. Why don't you put it out." So it was each cigarette rather than my habit that he confronted. I felt like I had to make the accommodations because he was being so honest and so personal. He wasn't saying anything about me. He wasn't saying, "It's really bothering me and my air. Why are you doing that?" He just said, "That hurts my lungs." What could I say? I really was good about not smoking around him. If he would have come out and directly attacked me, that would have set fires.

I've come to know that smoking is a screen between people. I'm really much more spontaneous now. I don't have to plan for ashtrays and other equipment. I'm freed from that.

Smoking is so vicious. It's a crippling, debilitating addiction. I've learned how really fragile

188

we are. When I see a guy on a lung machine who's still smoking, I understand. I'm always just one drink or one cigarette from being crazier than a bedbug. Because of what I've been through, I feel more with humanity than separate from it. I have lived through some bad times with both smoking and drinking. I think with my history, and where I'm sitting today inside of this house, I've sure had some good luck. I'm living on the fuel of that feeling of lucking out, of missing a freight train, because I know I could still be smoking. I would have different friends. I would probably get a new husband. I would organize my life differently.

With quitting smoking, the replacement factor is really important. We must find whatever it is that will turn the spiritual pump. The Twelve Steps helped me. Taking the leap of faith into the Steps, and asking people how they quit and then trying to transpose the information so it was valuable to me, worked. Those Steps seem to work for me for everything. The more I get parts of myself in line, the better my life feels. So when I feel mad, I know I am able to act appropriately, or when I feel sad, or when I feel happy. My behavior has started to have some appropriateness; my perceptions match my environment. When I feel paranoid it's because I am in a dark alley, so to speak. I think working the Steps leads to congruency.

Being smoke-free positively affects relationships, especially for women. I don't know for men. For most women, relationships are so integral and have such a high value in our lives. It's harder and harder to smoke when we know that smoking is a screen. When I finally got through my withdrawal, I tapped into that faith that I really would come out on the other side. I didn't have faith the other five times I tried to quit.

I believe there are people who will go right to their end smoking and it's not their fault because it's not willpower, nor is it because they didn't work the Steps right. I think maybe it's just fate. More and more I believe in some "recycling" process, not reincarnation, but some process that makes some sense for why people go through their lives not having the blessings others have. Why can some people quit when they are 70, and some like my dad, quit at 60, and why did I get off when I was 30? It's hard to explain. It seems that all of us are given the choice to make the best of our opportunities. Some of us will. That's my philosophy in a nutshell.

KATHY

*Age 46. Divorced mother of four, ages
17 to 26; sells real estate; loves tennis,
people, traveling, and art history.*

I don't remember my very first cigarette but I
do remember that at the time James Dean was
popular and I was about fifteen. My dad smoked
Salems and Camels, and he kept them in a
drawer in our buffet. My brother Joe and I used
to steal those and go smoke them out behind the
garage. Because I hated Salems, I began to buy
my own. First I smoked Pall Malls and somewhere along the way the Marlboro man got me.
It got to be cool to smoke Marlboros.

I really liked smoking and it seemed everybody
did it. For sure all my friends did. In actuality, a
lot of kids probably didn't smoke. Everybody
tried it but not everyone kept it up. At slumber
parties if one person had a pack of cigarettes everybody smoked, but not everybody started buying them after that.

My sister, Rita, was one of the kids who didn't
smoke. We shared a third-floor bedroom and I
can remember sitting and smoking and blowing
the smoke out the window, and threatening her
with decapitation if she told on me. Even though
I smoked with regularity, I never smoked around
my parents until after I got married. (I may even
have had my first child before I smoked in front
of them even though they both smoked.) I was
afraid they would shame me for smoking so I
didn't risk it. I didn't swear around my parents

either. I didn't do anything around my parents except be absolutely darling. It was my little sisters that got to be brats. I guess I was terrified that they would abandon me or something, so I was always on my good behavior.

I can recall when I made the decision that I was old enough to smoke in front of my mother. I remember actually lighting up at her house and feeling both defiant and self-conscious, but nothing really happened. There weren't any negative repercussions. I was 20 or 21 by that time. I always treated my dad like he was stupid, so I just smoked in front of him and figured if he said anything to me I would just pretend like he already knew I smoked. If he confronted me, I planned to say, "Well, you know I smoke. What's your problem?"

I enjoyed smoking. I loved it from the very first time. When I was about 21 or 22 and pregnant with my second child, I tried to quit smoking and realized then that I was hooked. I couldn't quit and that surprised me. I hadn't tried to quit because I was pregnant. I just decided to quit; however, I can remember making the decision not to quit after all. It was a Saturday and my husband was at work. By four o'clock in the afternoon, I was in tough shape. I was really impatient with my year-and-a-half-old daughter because I was crazy from withdrawal. I needed a cigarette badly. We had only one car so I had to wait for Tom to get home. When he got there, I was sitting on the front step with Chris and jumped in the car, drove to the store and bought a pack of cigarettes. That was the first time I ever was aware that I couldn't quit just anytime I wanted.

I tried to quit a few more times after that because of the consequences smoking was causing. I burned holes in clothes and furniture. Oftentimes it was because I'd drink too much. I remember one time burning a hole in a brand-new, gorgeous dress when I was drunk. It never occurred to me to quit drinking, but I did try to quit smoking several times. I'd never last more than a day and then I'd decide the hole wasn't that bad and I'd go buy a pack of cigarettes. I continued to smoke pretty consistently for the next twenty years.

Early in my smoking history, I was confronted by the tragic effects of smoking because my mother-in-law had cancer and the doctors made her quit smoking. She had a breast removed even. And yet, neither my husband nor she suggested I quit. But the consciousness, the whole awareness of the real danger of smoking was low then. And at that time, most everybody I associated with smoked. All my family, my parents, and friends, too, all except my husband. Actually I was surprised recently to read statistics that showed only one-third of the population smoked. I figured it was the other way around.

Even though I had quit a day, here and there many times, I never seriously worked on quitting until after I was divorced and in a relationship with a man who hated smoking. I was terrified that if I smoked in front of him, he would abandon me. That was my direct motivation to quit.

Also, at the time, I had a neighbor who had a real husky voice. Her doctor had been on her for years to quit smoking. She even had polyps on her throat. That motivated me too. Additionally, a friend and traveling companion who was allergic to cigarette smoke influenced me. Our agreement always was that I'd never smoke in our room when we were on a trip together. And normally that worked out okay because we would travel to places that were warm, like Florida and Mexico, where I could go out on the balcony and smoke. So my smoking was never really a problem, not until we planned a 30-day trip to Europe in January when it was going to be cold. I knew I was going to feel real resentful about having to go down to the lobby of the hotel or out in the hallway or somewhere to smoke. I loved traveling with her and I really loved our friendship. I didn't want to feel resentful. I knew I had to quit smoking to go on the trip or I would end up hating her. Fortunately, while planning the trip, I got more heavily involved with John and decided to quit, even before the trip departure. But it wasn't easy.

It was awful. Every time I've quit, it's gotten worse, too. The withdrawal is absolutely horrible. The first three days are horrible and then the ninth, tenth, and eleventh days are real hard again, and then at six weeks it's terrible again. At the time, one of my sisters was quitting too. We were going to college together, and we'd sit in the smoking room and smoke and then she'd eat a whole tube of toothpaste before she'd go home and see her husband. She told me it's normal to grieve the loss of cigarettes and that the sixth week and the sixth month and then anniversary dates are the hardest times in the grief process. If you're aware of that beforehand, you can watch out for those times and get over the humps.

The second time I quit it was really hard around the six-week period too. But in general I continued to miss cigarettes anyway, no matter how long I had been off. Today is my seventeenth month anniversary for not smoking and that's the longest I've ever gone without a cigarette. Fourteen-and-a-half months was the longest I had ever quit prior to this time. But I still miss cigarettes, not all the time, but occasionally.

My form of quitting each time was by toughing it out, and the rewards have never been particularly great. I know it's delusional but it seems my consequences for smoking were not as severe as they are for not smoking. While smoking I'd have less breath on the tennis court, but since quitting smoking I've gained so much weight that I have as much trouble getting around a tennis court as I did 40 pounds ago while smoking a pack-and-a-half of cigarettes a day. My lungs are pinker, but my rewards for being a nonsmoker are not great.

When I quit the time before this one and went fourteen-and-a-half months smoke-free, I missed smoking every single day and finally, one day I called up my sister and told her I was going to start smoking again. I asked her if she would still love me and she said "yes." She suggested I wait a few hours before going out to buy cigarettes. I did but went out and bought cigarettes anyway. This was during a period of my life when I was trying to control my drinking. I would slip into drinking every once in awhile after two or three weeks of sobriety, and I believed that if I smoked it would be easier to quit drinking. Of course that wasn't true. I felt shame for having let people down. Some good friends had really supported my not smoking. My traveling companion used to bring me flowers on my monthly anniversaries. She had been so excited when I quit smoking. She was real disappointed. It was easy to feel defensive but I was manufacturing the shame. Nobody shamed me but I managed to feel it anyway.

I smoked again for about two-and-a-half years. And then I started going out with another man who didn't smoke. One night we were playing Trivial Pursuit with a crowd and I was the only smoker. I felt real uncomfortable and that night was the last time I smoked. By then I was sober too. I'd been going to A.A. for a year-and-a-half and I hadn't had a drink for about six or eight months. But, in the meantime, I had skin cancer. The doctor kept telling me to quit smoking. He said he'd rather I expose my body to the heaviest megarays of sun for the rest of my life than to smoke. He told me he could carve skin cancer out of me for ever and ever and ever, but he couldn't carve my lungs out. That scared me, but not enough to quit right away.

Finally, the combination of the information,

experience, and a date who didn't smoke gave me the strength to quit again, but it was total insanity. I was going to real estate school and it was pretty stressful. I'd been out of college for a while and there I was, sitting in classes and taking tests while in withdrawal. To this day I can't believe I survived that without smoking. I quit smoking on a Tuesday and took the real estate test on Saturday. I studied, and prayed, "God, if You intend for me to be a nonsmoker, I'm going to pass the test." But I couldn't concentrate. My concentration was totally gone. I could barely get through a *People* magazine. I couldn't watch television or read. When I discovered I could get all the way through a *People* magazine without jumping up off the couch 500 times, I knew I was making progress.

I just couldn't sit still. I was in constant motion, mostly from my chair in the living room to the refrigerator. One of the reasons I had always started smoking again after quitting earlier times was because I gained so much weight. Before going to treatment for alcoholism I gained 30 pounds. I went to treatment as a nonsmoker and started smoking about two weeks later. I couldn't deal with all the pain going on with me, and everybody there smoked. I really didn't want to start smoking again but I was so preoccupied with it. One of the counselors said the decision to start again was between me and my Higher Power. I went right back to my room and took a pack of my roommates' cigarettes and started smoking. The 30 pounds I'd gained haunted me and I was desperate to lose the weight. Every time I tried to diet I'd go crazy. I'd just crawl out of my skin. Going back to smoking then was actually helpful. I was able to stay on a diet and not feel like I was going to crawl out of my skin.

What I know now is that nicotine is a mood-altering chemical that keeps my fear level manageable. So once again I smoked for fourteen months and I loved every minute of it, knowing full well that I was going to quit again someday when I got a little bit more sobriety. My A.A. sponsor also really encouraged me to get some more sobriety and to trust that when I was ready to quit I would know it. And that was what I did.

I was surprised when I actually quit. A friend of mine had just been diagnosed with lung cancer. He was my age and he had only months to live. I was going on a trip the day I heard about him and I made a decision to quit when I got home from my trip. I didn't even wait until I got home. The day that I left to come home, I quit. I'd gone out to play tennis about eleven o'clock and I couldn't even see the ball. Withdrawal had set in. But I was done. I sat in the no-smoking section on the way home and I haven't had a cigarette since.

I had been through quitting a lot of times before, so I knew what to expect, but it was even worse than I remembered it. Fortunately, a friend spoon-fed me a lot of good information. She had quit about three months earlier. I got her program on a one-to-one basis. It was really nice;

it was helpful. She would tell me physically what was happening to me. She had a medical background and explained how nicotine was a toxin, a poison, and that was why my body was just crawling.

She really hand-held me throughout this period. Another woman my age who had quit several months before really supported me, too. Also I swam every day, sometimes two or three times a day. I took a lot of whirlpools and bubble baths during the first three or four days. And I went for a massage every other day for the first week, plus I didn't eat sugar. The first three days were really horrible. My ears rang. My skin crawled. I felt like I was going to come right out of my skin. It was a horrible withdrawal. Having people around, telling me that it would get better, helped. The other thing that really helped a lot was reading my daily meditation books and substituting the word "cigarettes" for "alcohol." And I used affirmations over and over and over again.

I truly believed in my heart that God's will for me was that I would be a nonsmoker. I had gone to an effective living seminar three or four years before where they taught us how to use affirmations for more successful living. They had very specifically suggested that if you are still smoking, and would like to be a nonsmoker, you could create affirmations about being a nonsmoker and repeat them daily. Their theory was that your subconscious doesn't know the difference between past, present, and future. It can only hear what it is given. It doesn't act on it in any kind of a time frame. I used my nonsmoking affirmations for two or three months, even before I actually quit smoking. That may have been the catalyst, along with my friend's death. At any rate, one day I knew I was done with smoking.

The second phase of not smoking for me is a craving for tobacco that's really tied in with my addiction to sugar. I get the nicotine withdrawal symptoms when I go on a sugar binge and my thinking gets all screwed up. I rationalize that if I could smoke, the sugar withdrawal would go away. Sugar bingeing causes the crawling skin, the ringing ears, and the inability to deal with reality — all the same symptoms that occur with tobacco withdrawal. I don't understand it, but I sit in my bed and I know that if I smoke, my discomfort will go away. Instead, I choose to go to Superamerica and buy donuts or something.

My struggle may never be over. Just the other day my craving hit. I left work. I was parked in the underground garage. I came off the elevator and could tell someone had been smoking in the hallway. I smelled the cigarettes and had a euphoric memory of how I loved smoking. By the time I got to my car (which was maybe a hundred feet from the place where I smelled the cigarette smoke), I had already thought about stopping at the Superamerica near work to buy a pack of cigarettes. I didn't want to smoke in my brand-new car, but I figured I could just smoke a cigarette kind of, like around the edges, just smoke a half of one and throw it away. The first one doesn't taste very good anyway. In my fantasy, I figured that when I got home, I could hide them from my daughter. I knew she was working. I figured I could quit the next day. I knew it would be real painful, but I could do it. I hadn't even reached my car and this whole scenario had gone through my head. It really hit me just what an addict I really am. I don't even want to smoke, but that's just how quickly the craving can hit.

In order to quit I really needed the affirmations for strength. I still use them. The one I use the most is: "God's will for me is that I am a nonsmoker." I truly believe in that affirmation, and it feels good. It was probably the first real direct conscious contact with a Higher Power I've ever had in all the years I've been in a Twelve Step program. I also used an affirmation about abundance. This one still helps me when I get into abusive overeating. "There's abundance in the world and I have more than enough." This affirmation has to do with filling the inner hole that smoking or food or whatever takes care of.

After seventeen months and lots of struggling, I'm really glad I'm a nonsmoker, mostly because it gets more and more difficult all the time to smoke and enjoy it. I was at a brunch recently with seventeen women and there were two smokers there and no ashtrays! It just wasn't acceptable to smoke. More and more people want their homes to be smoke-free.

Going to a restaurant with eight people and being the only smoker is not easy either. I'm really glad that I don't have to put up with that anymore. It feels good to go some place for four or five hours and not have to leave because I have to go smoke. I no longer have to stand around with all the icky people at a party because they're surrounding the only ashtray.

And I assume I'm getting healthier, although I don't necessarily feel better physically. It's wonderful to wake up in the morning without that terrible taste in my mouth, but I only noticed that change in the first few weeks after quitting; since then, I don't remember what the terrible taste is like. I forget what cigarette hangovers are like, too. It's nice not to have them, but I don't think about it very often.

I've gained 40 pounds and it's real hard not to focus on that as a direct result of being a non-smoker. But the reality is that I have a problem with substance abuse, and right now my substance is food. I joined a group for food substance abusers last week and that feels good. I think I'm on the homestretch.

I know that I'm a nonsmoker forever. I still think about smoking whenever I have agitation. Whenever I have anxiety, I want to smoke because it used to take down my anxiety level. But I can't think of anything that would make me so anxious that I would believe smoking could cure it. I have other ways to deal with my anxieties now.

STRENGTH THROUGH MEDITATION

STRENGTH THROUGH MEDITATION

The stories you have just completed reading were told to me by men and women like yourself. These are men and women for whom the struggle to give up nicotine, in order to become their better selves, was not an easy decision. Nor was it easy to remain loyal to this commitment. All of them admitted to needing support from friends or from a Higher Power or both in order to get through the unexpectedly difficult days or particularly trying circumstances that occasionally arose. Each of them might have found the struggle less formidable had they been privy to the series of meditations that follow.

Millions of people, specifically those who are enjoying the support and friendship offered in Twelve Step programs like Alcoholics Anonymous, Al-Anon, and Narcotics Anonymous,* have grown to love and depend upon the spiritual guidance offered in daily meditation books.

The purpose of these books** is to offer quiet and very personal support, edification as well as insight and hope to the individual who really wants a better life. The following 90 meditations are offered for the same purpose.

---

*There are over 100 different kinds of Twelve Step programs active at the present time throughout the world.

**Such as *Twenty-Four Hours a Day, Each Day a New Beginning, The Promise of a New Day, Touchstones,* and *Night Light* — all available from Hazelden Educational Materials.

I settled on a series of 90 meditations because most people find the first three months after quitting nicotine the most difficult. And it's during these first three months that we're most vulnerable. It's imperative we remember we're only a cigarette away from being ensnared once again in the clutches of tobacco. Having a brief passage to read when we're feeling insecure about our resolve to not smoke will get us over the hump, beyond the urge to smoke. We can quietly turn to the same meditation or a different one as many times as we'd like throughout the day. The urges will pass, I promise you. And the meditations will offer strength. This, too, I promise you.

If you are still not as comfortable a nonsmoker as you had hoped for at the end of 90 days, begin again with reading Day 1. Many of us who read other daily meditation books read and reread the same books throughout a lifetime. Each day, a meditation we've read many times before will offer us new insight and additional strength because we will have grown and changed since our last reading of it.

The quotes introducing each meditation were spoken to me by those interviewed. They inspired my thoughts as I wrote the meditations. It's my prayer that you will find comfort, guidance, strength, and, most of all, hope in the days ahead by reading the pages that follow. Remember, whatever our goal happens to be, all of us need support to meet with success. Let the meditations give you that support. Let them carry you forward to the triumph that awaits you.

Day 1

"I don't have to quit forever; I can go back and use tobacco tomorrow if I want to; all I have to do is just not use it today."

We can do anything for this one day. Nothing will be too much for us. We can even break the day down into each of its 24 hours if the struggle demands it. We can then focus on just one hour at a time. Assuredly, we can survive 60 minutes at a time without a cigarette. How freeing it is to realize we only have to quit smoking for today.

It's helpful to remember all we are ever guaranteed is the present. We can hope for a fruitful future. And most likely it will come to pass; however, each time we give our attention to "when" rather than now, we're missing the richness of the tapestry our experiences are weaving.

Our decision to not smoke today, coupled with both the pain and the glory of our choice, will add to the meaning and the beauty of our tapestry. Today is our gift from the Creator. How we live these 24 hours is our gift in return.

I will do whatever I need to, to live without a cigarette today. It's all the life I'm certain of.

"I realized I really was powerless and trusted that if other people could do it, so could I."

Nicotine is powerful, so powerful. It has had me in its grip for a long time and it doesn't easily let go. My compulsion to smoke can't be controlled and it haunts me. But the decision to give in to the compulsion is controllable — by me, every time it comes. I am only powerless over the desire, not the decision to smoke.

My struggle to live without tobacco feels lonely and painful, but millions have survived it before me; millions are living through it with me, today. I am strengthened by knowing we share these moments in time. We are bonded even though we are strangers to one another.

I feel stronger just knowing I'm sharing this struggle with a friend I'll never meet.

"I can manage the withdrawal. It will come and I trust it will go away."

Every moment has its time. Pleasurable moments with a friend as well as painful moments because of hurt feelings pass very quickly. I must remember the adage "this too shall pass" when the desire to smoke again clouds my thoughts and disrupts my actions.

The moments that herald the euphoric recall of a day's first cigarette are just as fleeting as the moments I'll spend at a stop sign or dialing a phone today. Time passes on. I can't stop it, nor does it wait for me. My desire to smoke today will pass because its moment will pass. All I have to do is give my attention to the next moment as it signals me.

I can live through today's collection of moments without tobacco.

*"One problem is I don't ask for help
when I want a cigarette."*

Why do I think I must do everything alone?
Am I ashamed to say I need help? Am I afraid I'll
look weak if I admit how very hard it is to quit?

No smoker finds it easy to quit. Some do it
without much fanfare, but not without some inner struggle. It's much better to get support from
friends and co-workers who will want to help us
stay committed to our decision to stop.

Whenever we share ourselves freely with someone else, particularly when we're revealing how
vulnerable we are, or how the present struggle is
difficult, we'll know a new freedom and a new
closeness to the friend who has listened. Everyone likes to offer help; when we ask for help during these difficult times, we're doing something
valuable for two people — ourselves and the one
whom we ask.

*Let me remember that my asking for help today
is a gift to someone else, too.*

*"Just one day is all I have to quit for,
and they'll add up."*

There is no doubt we can do anything asked of us and survive any hardship or trauma for just one day. And what a good fortune that this is all our Higher Power has ever expected of us. Little by little, our experiences unfold by design — this is all the better to learn our lessons by.

Quitting smoking is just another unfolding experience, and we have only today to focus on. No matter how enticing a cigarette may seem, regardless of the depth of our longing, we can abstain today. And tomorrow will take care of itself.

For many of us, past attempts at quitting were thwarted because we envisioned years of tomorrows, feeling deprived of the comfort we sought from cigarettes. How helpful it is to quiet our minds to the future. It isn't here, now. Only today is here — 24 short hours, a mere flash. Surely we can survive a mere flash without a cigarette.

I'll look at today — only today, and I know I can live without smoking.

"For most people, quitting is not just black and white; for most people, it's a series of stopping and starting and stopping again."

The decision to quit must be renewed daily. It's hard to give up the friend who comforted us when we were scared or sad — who never deserted us when we were lonely, keeping us company during a long evening at home or on the road traveling.

Let's not ignore our grief. It's normal and healthy to grieve the loss of something that was as close as our breath. But let's also remember cigarettes were dangerous friends; our personal welfare was forever at stake while in their company.

One day at a time, even one hour at a time is all we need to concern ourselves with. Let's decide now, for the rest of today only, that we will not smoke. Our tomorrows will take care of themselves.

It will strengthen me to recommit myself to this decision every day. Twenty-four hours is such a short span in contrast to all that has gone before.

*"It's wonderful not being in conflict
with my values anymore."*

For a long time I didn't want to smoke, and yet
I did. I'd feel ashamed I couldn't just quit. At
night I'd resolve to quit, but start again the next
morning. What a relief it is knowing I'm not
unique.

Values are what guide our thoughts and
actions. When we're in conflict with our values,
we feel self-conscious and ill-at-ease. Values can't
be ignored, though we try to pretend otherwise.
Pain and shame are frequent reminders that our
values are alive and demanding our attention.

If I decide to smoke again, my values will torment me, and I can't quiet them. But I can make
the right decision about how I'll live my life today, a decision that promises peacefulness
throughout my being.

*My values love me, sometimes more than I love
myself.*

"I started doing some imaging of myself as a nonsmoker."

Our minds are so powerful. We can prepare ourselves for a challenge by visualizing ourselves gracefully surviving it. We can get help for working through a tense situation with a friend or foe by imaging the encounter in a positive light. Imaging, in a detailed way, how we might handle any experience will give us the courage and the strength to tackle whatever confronts us.

Using imagery will deepen our commitment to being a nonsmoker. In time, we'll not be able to imagine we ever smoked. However, in the meantime, we'll be helped by systematically spending some time alone, quietly meditating on an image of ourselves going through the hours of the day, and happily acting out our part, without the hindrance of a cigarette.

Imagery works because it can make something we haven't yet experienced seem familiar. It teaches us how to act in the experience visualized. We quickly become "old hands" because our minds have made us experienced.

My experience as a nonsmoker will be enhanced by a few moments of imagery today.

Day 9

> *"I would buy a pack of cigarettes and smoke two. And then I'd stand over the toilet and rip them all up and flush the toilet. And then the next day I'd do something similar."*

Tobacco's power is awesome when we give in to it. We all have memories, strong and awful memories of behavior for which we feel shame. Maybe it's digging through trash for a cigarette butt that's long enough for one puff, or stealing change from a child's piggy bank for that late night trek to the all-night store for a needed smoke.

Today, we want freedom from the pull of tobacco. That's why we're here now. We want to be in charge of our own lives, of our own decisions regarding time, money, health, and activities. If we're smoking, we're not in charge. Tobacco is king, and we're only its subjects, bowing to its many demands.

I don't have to create more awful memories for myself today. Rather, I can create ones that will continue to give me hope and strength.

"Quitting smoking and quitting drinking are just the first steps for me. I feel excited about my future at last."

Each day stretches before us, awaiting our involvement. Whether we approach our activities at work or home with enthusiasm or dread depends on the attitude we've cultivated. Attitudes don't just happen; they are honed ever so carefully, and they are nourished by us every moment.

When we've made a radical change in our lives, one that we know nourishes us beneficially, it lends an air of excitement to our perception of the activities that lay ahead. The future can always excite us. And it will as long as we are committed to being the people we really want to be, and remain open to the adventure each day promises.

Becoming a nonsmoker is our chance to be the person we long to be. New doors will open to new opportunities because we have closed the door on the self who controlled us in years past. All of life — play, work, friends, talents, and dreams — will take on a new appearance now that we can see with a clearer vision.

Not smoking has changed how everything looks to me. It's almost like being reborn. Life feels fresh, like the air in early spring.

Day 11

"I am changing my patterns. I'm taking control. The nicotine is no longer in control, and that feels good."

There are so many activities we thought we'd never be able to do without the company of a cigarette. Most of us were convinced smoking helped us think, relax, write, and converse. Probably, we relied on cigarettes when we were lonely or afraid. And now there's genuine joy in the discovery that we can get through the stressful as well as the menial tasks that demand our attention during the day without the assistance of a cigarette.

Making changes in our lives, changes we're certain are beneficial to us in the present as well as the future, feels really good. We do have the power and the responsibility for our personal development. We have always had them; but in many instances, we didn't make good decisions about our behavior. However, quitting smoking has given us a very strong taste of self-determination in action, and it's exhilarating.

We'll discover as time goes on that it will get increasingly easier to make other healthy choices for ourselves. And each beneficial choice we make will strengthen us for the next.

I can do anything asked of me today without a cigarette.

"If I'm in a certain situation where I know I would have smoked in the past, I'm removing myself from that situation."

The memories of how, when, and where we smoked are terrifically powerful, particularly in the early weeks of our abstinence. Memories tug at us, grabbing our attention; they tempt us, and they distract reality. We can't trust the fond recall of cigarettes over coffee. The real truths — the coughing and congestion, the stains and burns on our bodies and clothes, the frequent searches for leftover butts long enough to smoke — are too easily hidden from our thoughts.

Fortunately, through choice, we can avoid certain situations, activities, or people that seemed to compel us to smoke in the past. We need not stay anywhere that doesn't nurture our new identity. We should only frequent places and spend time with people that will lovingly nurture our developing self. Each time we leave a setting that tempts us to smoke again, we'll grow in strength and self-esteem.

If I don't want to slip into my old habits, I'll avoid the slippery places today.

<u>Day 13</u>

"I feel better knowing I'm in control of something rather than being controlled. That gives me strength."

We can't control the weather, other people, or the outcome of most situations; but we can control our own behavior and attitude. We can either be contented nonsmokers or frustrated, nervous, and disgruntled ones. The choice is ours. The ability to control our thoughts and actions exists solely within ourselves; it's empowering to know we are in control of how we will behave today.

No friend or stranger in our path today can make us act against our will. We might be tempted to lash out, to feel shame or intimidation by another's behavior. But how we respond to any situation is totally within our control. It's an awesome responsibility taking charge of our lives, owning our behavior. And it's also inspiring and exhilarating.

I'm not smoking today because I am choosing this path for me. It's my decision and my life. I'm in charge!

"When the urge to smoke surfaces, I recognize it and let it pass."

Approximately every eight minutes, a smoker's body cries out for nicotine; and within minutes, the craving is generally satisfied. We should not be surprised that our bodies are experiencing torment and letting us know about it. Nicotine is a demanding and deadly drug, and it expects to imprison us once again. A strong urge is nicotine's bait.

We have some tools to handle the urges so they need not overwhelm us. We can very simply replace the thought with one that's more beneficial to us. We are the creators of all our thoughts. Negative thoughts don't happen to us — we give them birth.

We can develop the skill of imaging and, in our mind's eye, see a picture of us contentedly going about our daily affairs smoke-free. We can also turn to others who, like us, are opting for a healthier life without cigarettes. Support is always available. And finally, we each have a Higher Power who comforts, guides, and eases our path when we're on the right track.

I am on the right track today. I'll let all the forces help me stay on this track.

> *"This last time I quit, it was easier be-*
> *cause I wanted to quit. I didn't have*
> *the leftover feeling that I ought to*
> *quit."*

Relapse has been a reality for many of us. Nic-otine is a formidable drug, and it gives us a tough battle. If it's a battle we've lost in the past, per-haps it's because we were trying to quit for some-one else or because we entered the fight alone without the support or strength available to us from our Higher Power or our network of friends and other nonsmokers.

We don't ever have to rely solely on our own resources to accomplish any goal, to shift our per-ceptions, or to make a major change in our lives. Our own resources are seldom enough. They are strengthened many times over when we team them with the strength of friends who want us to succeed and with a Higher Power that is loving. This decision not to smoke is no harder than we make it.

I'm at will to look within myself and to others to help me adhere to my decision today.

*"Right now I still feel out of control
because I'm not smoking."*

Tobacco was the object of our attention. Buying it, stashing it, hoarding it, using it, and even on occasion hiding it. We were in control over our relationship with tobacco, which provided a false sense of security. Our need to feel in control of something — situations, personal achievements, other people — is awesome and yet thwarted on most occasions. Tobacco filled the need for control, and now that's gone.

Our decision to quit smoking is giving us an opportunity to recognize the emptiness of false security. One lesson is the only control that rests securely with us is the control we express over our behavior and our attitude.

There's another lesson if we want to explore it — it's a spiritual lesson. It rests with our acknowledgment of a greater power within us, a power that will guide our behaviors and soften our attitudes. Turning to the power within will offer us the security we longed for from tobacco.

Today will be restful and productive if I turn within for security.

> *"Since I quit smoking, I can't concentrate."*

It's not unusual to be obsessed with the desire to smoke. Smoking was a key part of nearly every activity that involved us. When a best friend moves away, our thoughts are drawn to that person often. A gentle reminder to return our attention to the present is really all that's necessary, but let's not be surprised by the frequency of this necessity.

How resilient human beings are. There's very little we can't recover from. And we can recover from smoking. Problem solving may be harder for a while. A superior novel may not quite captivate us. Even a scintillating conversation may lose our attention — but time is very healing.

If we truly desire freedom from our addiction to tobacco, we must be patient with ourselves. The obsession to smoke will leave us. Our ability to concentrate will return without the distraction that accompanied smoking.

I'll not dwell on my hunger for cigarettes today. It's merely a thought and I'm in charge of my thoughts.

"I feel good about myself for being able to stay away from cigarettes for 22 years."

Even one day without cigarettes feels like a milestone when we first quit. And it is! We deserve congratulations for our efforts. It's appropriate for us to share our success with someone who can understand our struggle and who can give us support.

Remember, we have only one day at a time to not smoke. We can make the decision anew tomorrow. Today is all we have. Perhaps someday we'll also have 22 years of one days of not smoking. But for now, there isn't any experience we can't survive, even the torment of no cigarette, for this one day.

At today's end, how proud and grateful we'll feel about not succumbing to the frequent urges to smoke. The people who quit for one or ten or twenty-two years aren't endowed with any special characteristics. They are just like ourselves, but they're more comfortable with their choice to not smoke.

I can easily handle today without a cigarette if I rely on my inner strength and the support of well-wishers.

Day 19

*"Everybody becomes a nonsmoker
during the night."*

Tackling the challenge of giving up cigarettes
seemed monumental at first until we were reminded that we survived six to eight hours every
night with no tobacco. True, those hours were
uncluttered by the tension of deadlines or angry
people or unfamiliar situations. But the important point is we have survived years of nighttimes
without smoking. It's a fact worth rejoicing.

When the urge to resume the habit tempts us,
it's strengthening to remember those accumulated hours of not smoking. Any technique we
can employ to strengthen our commitment is well
worth the effort. Let's be mindful that there are
very few activities more harmful to ourselves,
and to those forced to experience our polluted
air, than smoking.

Let's live these next 24 hours one at a time, as
willing nonsmokers. The 8 hours we're asleep
will take care of themselves, leaving only 16 for
us to be in charge of. One hour at a time is manageable.

*I can easily handle a 60-minute segment. It's re-
ally pretty easy to string a few of them together.*

"Since quitting, I've felt like I'm in a honeymoon period. I'm real positive."

Taking charge of our lives — whether through a new job, leaving a bad relationship, or changing our eating or drinking habits — is a guaranteed way to boost our self-esteem. Each time we follow through on a decision destined to benefit us either spiritually, physically, or emotionally, we find instantaneous gratification. We are learning that quitting smoking offers just such gratification.

Though it's not easy for all of us to do, saying no to tobacco this moment feels good and right because we are taking back our personal power. Nicotine no longer controls our thoughts, our attitudes, our behaviors. We are discovering just how much time we devoted to smoking. The irony is that smoking not only took minutes and hours away from each day's activities, but months, perhaps years from our expected life span. Tobacco, in any form, is double jeopardy.

I look in the mirror today and I feel great. I'm excited about taking charge of my behavior.

> *"It's really special I care enough about myself that I don't want to kill myself."*

For many years, most of us have been in a state of denial about the harmful effects of cigarettes. Physical problems have even been indicators for some of us, but we shook off the reality. Yet, here we are. At last! To the relief of family and friends, we are living one day at a time without nicotine.

It wasn't an easy decision to give up our crutch; smoking had coaxed us through many long nights and troubling experiences. But our return had diminished greatly: nicotine eventually takes its toll on every user because users become abusers; few — ever so few — are social smokers. Seemingly, there's an addict lurking in everybody. Our drug of choice varies — that's all.

Even though we're in the early phase of freedom from nicotine, it's essential to congratulate ourselves for opting to live rather than participate in a slow, passive death. We have many brothers and sisters who need our example.

It's never too early to congratulate myself on my progress.

"Whenever the urge to smoke came over me the first few days, I used a little mental trick of pretending I was between cigarettes."

There are thousands of techniques we can use to support our efforts not to smoke, and we should not shy away from any of them. Nobody finds stopping easy; we often have to give ourselves permission to be honest about the difficulty we're experiencing.

Too many of us grew up with the advice, "Be tough. It's weak to need help." The reality is that asking for help strengthens rather than weakens us, and the people we ask for help are strengthened as well. Shared vulnerability enhances the spiritual development of all who are privy to the sharing.

Imaging ourselves as healthy, happy, contented nonsmokers helps to reprogram the subconscious; thus, it's a valuable tool in our reeducation process. Simply acknowledging each urge and letting it pass can also become a useful and easy habit to develop. Let's not forget that we are the maker of our thoughts. We can replace any urge with whatever thought we prefer.

I'm the master of my mind for all these 24 hours ahead of me.

> *"I intentionally carried a pack of cigarettes around with me the whole day because I wanted to make it clear to myself that what I was doing was a choice."*

Accepting responsibility for who we are and the progress we've made with our lives is a sign of maturity. It's far easier to blame parents or bosses or "the system" for our struggles and failings.

Having quit smoking is a mature act because it's a choice we've made for ourselves. For most of us it took a great deal of thought and preparation. Perhaps others encouraged us, and their continuing support will strengthen us; but we are on our own and must be fully accountable only to ourselves.

Not smoking is a major change in our lives; smoking was our companion in virtually every activity that engaged us. We'll feel abandoned for a time. Our span of attention will be intermittent. Our patience and tolerance will likely be tested. But more importantly, our health — emotionally, physically, and spiritually — will be enhanced. We'd do well to focus on these positive aspects.

As a nonsmoker, I'm guaranteed a healthier life. I'll work on my gladness today.

"I feel such an emotional sense of loss whenever I quit."

Smoking has comforted me. It's been a very attentive friend, always softening my sadness, relieving my loneliness. I feel naked, frustrated, empty, and edgy without a cigarette to rely on. I can't expect these first few days to be easy. And it's okay to grieve the loss of my friend.

Surviving the first cup of coffee, the first meal, the first phone call, the first major argument, the first weekend, the first good cry without a cigarette will give me the strength needed to survive other difficult times. We can keep track of our milestones as we complete them, and our strength and our resolve will grow. Each moment without a cigarette is helping me become a person with a future of choices I hadn't dreamed of before.

The loss I feel today will pass, of that I'm certain.

Day 25

> *"Smoking isn't handsome or beautiful or sophisticated. It's a lie to believe otherwise."*

As a teenager, I was fully convinced that dangling a cigarette from my mouth made me appear sexy. I wanted to be noticed, and I certainly noticed others who smoked with a certain flair. Delusions die hard. What I chose to ignore then and for many subsequent years was that smoking causes teeth to stain, smelly breath, burns in favorite shirts or sweaters, and clothes to smell like dirty ashtrays.

Smokers, with every puff, are making emphatic statements about themselves, their attitude toward life, their level of self-respect, and their respect for those of us sharing their space. It's helpful to remember that smokers, like we so recently were, are choosing to disregard our desire to enjoy clean air. They are selfishly unconcerned with our health and well-being, along with their own. Having opted for slow suicide, they unfortunately have foisted a similar fate on those of us who must breathe their air. Our example as a smoker who has quit is the most powerful statement we can make.

I will have opportunities today to set an example for someone else who really would like to quit. The decision to do so needs my support.

"I had to take quitting little by little."

Making the decision to stop using tobacco is the first step, and that we've done. But there are many additional steps in the process of quitting; we can only go forward one day at a time, one step at a time.

It's helpful if we renew our commitment to quitting every morning. It's also helpful if we turn within ourselves for the strength to move through the urges that will assuredly arise throughout the day, particularly at those times when, in the past, we eagerly relied on a cigarette to calm our nerves or to distract us from a painful moment.

We all know someone who did smoke but who doesn't anymore. Giving someone the opportunity to help us through these early weeks will strengthen each of us. It's a rare person who simply lays aside tobacco and goes forward with no regrets.

Let me feel no shame for my struggle today. It's a mighty and worthy endeavor to choose a life free from tobacco.

Day 27

> *"I soon learned that no urge ever lasts more than 30 seconds."*

Urges to smoke are so powerful. They obsess us momentarily and we feel crazy with desire. It's helpful to know that urges are normal and fleeting. All we need to do is let them go. They will run their course in a matter of moments, and our attention will be captured by another thought or a fresh situation.

Urges serve as strong reminders of the power of nicotine, but urges can be accepted as gifts that support our decision not to smoke. Our lives as smokers weren't our own. Tobacco was in control of our thoughts, our attitudes, and our behavior. Perhaps we'd forget the insidious control nicotine demands if it weren't for the reminders the urges offer us.

When an urge tempts me today, I'll be grateful for the reminder that nicotine does not easily give up its prey.

"Smoking is poison for my body. I need my body to live. I owe myself that respect."

I liked smoking. It was my friend and it comforted me, I thought. Only now do I realize smoking was an enemy in disguise — an enemy to my body, to the bodies of those people subjected to my smoking, and to the environment housing us all.

It's helpful imaging tobacco with a skull and crossbones. In these early days of quitting we need constant reminders of the danger inherent in smoking, to our lungs and hearts and to the lungs and hearts of others — whether friends, co-workers, or strangers. We are human bodies sharing this planet, and each of us has a responsibility for the preservation of all of us.

My physical body needs my loving attention, my care, and gentle nurturing in order for it to serve me fully today and my many days ahead.

Day 29

"The best part of not smoking is the freedom."

Cigarettes tied me down. Thinking, talking, dreaming, reading, driving — they all sought cigarettes as accompaniment. Some of us thought we'd not be able to do any of those things alone, without the companionship of a cigarette. Some days it's very hard to "go it alone."

And yet, we've got a few days of freedom from tobacco behind us. How good it feels to know that tobacco is no longer more powerful than we are. Today I will keep track of all the activities I'm enjoying without a cigarette or a pinch of tobacco.

How glad I am that I can sit here quietly, reading this meditation and not be in need of a cigarette.

"I had been putting off quitting for years. But now I've done it!"

There's generally a lot of planning and talk, along with a few false starts, before we are able to leave cigarettes alone. And that's all part of the process. There is no right way to quit. There are as many ways to quit as there are smokers who want to give up tobacco.

Self-talk to support the decision to quit is valuable because our subconscious tucks away all the information we feed it. Affirming we are happy nonsmokers, particularly on every occasion we'd have normally smoked a cigarette or two, will help to break the old pattern of behavior while at the same time create a new image of ourselves. We have tremendous power, personally, to determine who we want to be and to strengthen those traits that will foster the identity that best suits us.

I am happy not smoking. I savor the strength I feel from sticking to this decision.

> *"If it's possible to stop smoking for an hour, it's possible to stop smoking for good."*

This moment is all we have. It's all we'll ever have. Our yesterdays are gone; regardless of what they held for us, they are past and we survived them. All we can ever be sure of experiencing for the remainder of this life is what involves us right now. And right now, whether we're in turmoil or euphoria, we don't need a cigarette to survive.

The future is unknown and illusionary. Moment by moment, the future becomes our present and introduces us to exactly what we need to grow. We've been promised the strength to move through our particular moments, and cigarettes can neither hasten nor help us with the steps we'll need to take.

It's helpful to take an inventory of the various experiences we've had since stopping tobacco. Many of them were stressful; and yet we're here now, and we didn't need to smoke to get here. We've had fearful periods, too, and we didn't smoke. We're learning, day by day, that no experience is too much for us to handle without a cigarette, and every experience is offering us information to grow.

I've learned it is possible to stop smoking for an hour. Fortunately, our lives are just a very long collection of hours.

"Nonsmoking is so day-to-day. It's sometimes a minute-to-minute kind of new identity."

It's harder not to smoke some days. A frustrating encounter with a co-worker or an emotionally charged argument with a friend or lover makes us hunger for a cigarette. Cigarettes used to comfort us. Feeling our anger or hurt or fear is oftentimes painful and very draining. Sometimes we miss the quiet comfort and freedom that smoking gave us. Smoking seemed like a friend then.

If smoking tempts me today, I'll remember my growth as a person depends on knowing and feeling whatever feelings are triggered by the day's events. And I'll remember smoking was never really a friend. Rather, smoking stunted my growth; it took away my power to make healthy choices.

When the urge to escape from today's lessons comes, I'll be quietly thankful that in a saner moment I chose to quit tobacco.

> 'I literally looked myself in the mirror
> more than once and said, 'You are a
> nonsmoker, and you want to stay that
> way.' "

We need to employ many techniques to stay committed to our decision not to smoke. Tobacco, like alcohol, is cunning, baffling, and powerful. The desire to smoke "just one" won't be a rare desire. And if we've let down our guard against starting again, if we've gotten complacent about the strength of the addiction, then we are very vulnerable to the appeal of "just one."

We must ask for the support of other nonsmokers throughout our early "recovery" from smoking. We must be willing to live through frequent urges to smoke and accept our powerlessness over those urges. More importantly, we must be willing to take responsibility for who we are and who we want to be. Standing before a mirror and reminding ourselves of who we are is a powerful tool in this struggle for growth.

When the urge to smoke strikes, I can either be my own best friend or my own worst enemy.

"I'm a committed nonsmoker, and I love it part of the time. But not always. I really do see quitting as a process."

Most of us can't just quit one day and never touch tobacco again. We stop and start and stop and start. And, hopefully, we'll one day stop forever. Even when that day comes, we may not be contented nonsmokers. Some days the idea of a cigarette is appealing. Hopefully, we'll be able to remember that one cigarette will never be enough.

To not want to smoke and yet to love the thought of one cigarette is familiar thinking during these early weeks of tobacco-free living. Let's not be concerned with our confusion nor with our strong desire to smoke. Desire can't make us act against our will. It can only tempt and tease us. The decision to smoke is separate from the desire.

I'll seek support from friends if I'm wavering in my decision making ability today

*"I quit every day and then smoked
every day, too."*

The desire to smoke is so overpowering some
days. Every activity, every memory, every anticipated event seems to beg for a cigarette. But with
the help of friends who want us to quit, and the
help of our inner spirit who really does wish us
good health and freedom from this addiction, we
can move beyond the momentary cravings that
crowd us throughout a day.

We need not repeat past patterns where we
quit and then smoked again all too quickly. This
time can be different if we are prepared to respond differently to the urges to smoke.

*I look forward to living through an urge today,
with the help of friends, both internally and
externally.*

"After I first quit, I would begin a project or begin reading or doing something with my hands, but I couldn't stay at it for long."

Did cigarettes foster concentration? It's doubtful, but it may seem that way now as we're struggling with our preoccupation to smoke. It's no wonder that we can't complete our work. Our attention span is so sporadic. But our thoughts don't happen to us; we are in charge of them, and our obsessive thinking about cigarettes is directly attributable to ourselves, which means we can change the program whenever we desire. Fortunate indeed!

It's a powerful realization that we are in command of our thoughts as well as our feelings. But it might also terrify us because it lays at our feet full responsibility for whatever we dwell on, whatever we see in others, and whatever we feel in response to any experience engaging us. There can be no more blaming others for our own feelings or actions.

I'm in charge of my own movie reel today. I can enjoy the day fully if I so choose.

> *"I know what the addiction is; and I know if I smoke even one cigarette, I may not be able to give up smoking again."*

Wavering from our commitment to stop, for even one quick puff, is a choice we best not make. One cigarette looks so innocent; and yet for an addict, there is no such thing as only one. Giving in to the urge allows the addiction to take control. Most of us have had experience with our own loss of control myriad times before. Let's not forget our earlier failed attempts to stop; even more important, let's remember the many avenues of help available to us if we seek them.

Anybody is willing to listen for a moment if we're struggling with an urge today. And that will strengthen us. If we're feeling lonely and caught in fond recall of the comfort cigarettes seemed to offer, now is our opportunity to let a friend step into the void, thus making two people feel worthy and comforted.

It's possible to think of urges to smoke as gifts honoring our growth, providing we let the urge guide us toward others or to a Higher Power for strength. Isolating ourselves with an urge gives the urge undeserved power.

Some days will be easier than others without cigarettes. The tough days will bring us closer to others, and that's something to be grateful for.

"Since I've quit smoking, I'm no longer destroying my clothes and my furniture on a regular basis."

Smoking is such a dirty and dangerous habit. We'll never know how many children, women, and men have died as the result of someone's smoking. Houses burn down; cars are wrecked; lungs are destroyed. What a relief to no longer be contributing to the destruction cigarettes cause.

Those of us struggling to be nonsmokers need each other's support along with the support of our friends and family. Giving up our steady companion results in feelings of loneliness. It's time to strengthen our companionship with others who, like us, don't smoke. In the process, we will be setting a good example for someone else who may also want to try life as a nonsmoker.

I will remember I'm setting a positive example for someone else today.

> *"I realized I had gone through half a day without a cigarette, and I hadn't come apart at the seams; so I decided to keep going with it."*

Quitting seemed tentative initially. It was more of a hope than commitment for most of us. And what a surprise we had when we survived the first day — then the first week. Self-esteem began to build. "I can do it!" But we still hesitated to announce it too loudly — just in case.

Now, it's a few weeks later. Sometimes we feel like we're barely hanging on. The urges to smoke still come and we wonder why. The fond recall of smoking frequently overwhelms us; at times like these, let's not hesitate to ask for help from our friends.

Quitting a habit that has befriended us for years is very difficult. We truly can't, comfortably, do it alone. And that's okay. In fact, that's good. We all need to nurture our dependence on others for help. We weren't meant to live our lives in solitary confinement. Our resources for strength exist outside ourselves — from friends — as well as within.

Any day that I'm struggling, I pray I can remember to turn to my network of friends. We are in this life to help one another.

"I no longer wake up in the middle of the night and have to smoke a cigarette before I can get back to sleep."

Sleeping straight through a night has been one of the unexpected, pleasurable results of life without tobacco. In the early weeks of our recovery from tobacco use, we likely slept much more than usual. For many of us accustomed to waking in the night, perhaps we never connected sleepless spells with nicotine deprivation. But our bodies were attuned to the many hours without tobacco. More restful sleeping is just one of the many benefits gracing our nights and subsequent days now.

What a miracle it is to be living through every moment of every day without cigarettes. We're not free of the desire perhaps; nor are we always content with our decision to quit. It's normal for us to grieve the loss, and even feel occasional anger over the choice we've made to not smoke. Fortunately, we don't have to shoulder any of our feelings alone. We have other nonsmokers to turn to for support and understanding, and we have the strength of a Higher Power who is always available to us.

I'll remember the miracle of my freedom from tobacco all day long.

> *"When I finally got through my with-drawal, I tapped into the faith that I really would come out on the other side."*

There is no doubt that we will "come out on the other side." We will survive the arduous process of stopping smoking, even though some of our days have been very difficult and we've wanted so badly to smoke again. What a tantalizing thought to have "just one." But we must not forget that, for us, there's no such thing as "just one."

When this struggle feels overwhelming, let's remember we're not alone. On this very day, there are no doubt thousands, perhaps tens of thousands who likewise are choosing to become nonsmokers. Imagining a group of us cheering each other on will lessen our pain and lighten our dark moods.

Our attitude is awesomely powerful. We can use it to our advantage each time conditions tempt us to renege on our commitment to not smoke.

What a marvelous image a cheering group of nonsmokers makes. I'll visualize us many times today.

*"I suddenly realized I had actual con-
trol over how I felt."*

It's a strengthening awareness to know that
we, and we alone, are responsible for how we
feel. For years perhaps, we've wanted to blame
others. "He makes me so mad!" "She did it to me
again!" Ultimately, we have to accept full responsibility for how we feel. The most dire conditions can't get us down without our consent.
We are willingly, though maybe unconsciously,
opting for the anger, the depression, or the feelings of inadequacy that are troubling us today.

Without tobacco to muffle our feelings, we're
much more aware of how frequently we entertain destructive feelings. They chart our course of
action; and most often, it's a course that a more
thoughtful, peaceful mind wouldn't have
charted.

We can and should take conscious, careful control of our moods, our thoughts, and our actions.
Never are we puppets whose strings are being
manipulated by foes or friends. We are actors in
control of ourselves throughout every scene of
this play called life.

*I will consciously choose my feelings today. No
one is in charge but me!*

> *"There's absolutely no question smoking damages one's health."*

When the urge to smoke arises today, as it most likely will, it's helpful to remind ourselves that smoking kills men, women, and children. Not only will we be at risk for cancer, heart disease, and home fires if we smoke, we'll put those we care about most at risk, too. To not smoke is a decision and one that we might need to make over and over today as an urge beckons.

Most of us have known one person who has experienced surgery or at least hospitalization because of the effects of tobacco. We've all heard a horror story about the agonizing death of a cancer patient, but we've generally believed it couldn't happen to us. Choosing a smoke-free life won't guarantee our absolute safety, but not smoking is a pretty good insurance policy. Smoking does damage health — ours and our children's.

I'll be grateful for the gift I'm giving myself and my family today by not smoking.

*"My experience taught me that if you
really want to quit, just keep trying."*

It's disheartening to quit smoking and then begin again. We feel ashamed and angry, maybe
even depressed that we couldn't remain committed to our resolve. And, somewhat embarrass-
ingly, we probably even feel a little relief that the
struggle to not smoke is over, at least for a while.

Those of us reading these words are lucky. We
have made the decision, once again, to live a day
at a time without cigarettes. And this time can be
different. We can rely on support from friends
and other nonsmokers — people who genuinely
want to help us. Each time an urge to smoke
overcomes us, we can read this meditation again
and again throughout the day. We have permission to go to any length to not smoke — if that's
our choice.

We can be just as successful with not smoking
as we can be playing a clarinet, a game of tennis,
or a rubber of bridge. Practice is the key — practice and the willingness to experience the struggle.

*Today I'll remember the old adage that "practice
makes perfect."*

Day 45

*"Cigarettes were my companion, my
solace."*

Giving up anything we love —pie, chocolate,
liquor, or cigarettes — makes us feel deprived. So
it's not surprising we feel abandoned without our
cigarettes to comfort us. But we have the choice
to see our deprivation as an opportunity to seek
solace from the people in our lives — men and
women who are not simply surrounding us by
chance. They've been handpicked by our Higher
Power and theirs. Together, we have miles to go
and much to learn.

This design for our lives is mysterious, but it is
loving and promises us growth. We can trust that
we'll not be led astray; rather, we'll be introduced to all the experiences meant for our fuller
development. Meeting these experiences without
the false aid of cigarettes promises a clearer
understanding of their meaning.

Let's not deprive ourselves of all the beauty,
knowledge, and growth meant for us by giving
undue attention to the fleeting moments of deprivation we feel over the loss of tobacco.

*I'll look lovingly upon my network of friends to-
day and recognize they are not here by chance.*

*"Quitting cold turkey means changing
your whole attitude, and it'll never
happen overnight."*

Patience is indeed a virtue, one seldom pos-
sessed by people like us who still yearn for the
mysterious contentment offered by a cigarette.
We wanted to quit painlessly and to go on with
our lives unchanged. But everything has
changed, and the unfamiliarity of our surfacing
feelings brings little pleasure as we've defined it.
The power and the choice to redefine it rests with
us.

It's a time to be gentle with ourselves and to
reflect on the distance we've traveled since childhood, trusting we'll move through this period of
discontent with as much comfort as we decide to
muster. Quitting smoking was a major decision
and an even more demanding undertaking. Let's
be patient and tolerant of our inner upheaval.
Time will heal.

*I'll remind myself that patience will reward me
tenfold today. I'll realize the benefits in all my
tomorrows.*

Day 47

> *"One of the pluses of not smoking is I can play good racquetball. All of a sudden I feel I can play forever again."*

No more breathlessness from climbing a short flight of stairs. Even running to catch a bus is a possibility now. No longer are we embarrassed by incessant coughing that we, friends, and co-workers knew was from our smoking. In a matter of weeks we can see the evidence of healthy bodily changes. And the improvements have just begun.

It's human nature to discount these improvements in our physical condition. We quickly forget we used to always opt for an elevator rather than the stairs. But our bodies will continue to renew themselves even without our attention. We are more aware of our mental condition; our self-esteem is in an upward climb. We're proud and grateful we've taken back our power from nicotine. We can share our gratitude by helping someone else who wants to stop.

I didn't get free of my addiction alone. I'll be available to support someone who wants to follow my example today.

> *"Smoking is really an out-and-out statement that 'I don't care about myself.' I'm glad I'm not saying that anymore."*

Smoking was glamorous or sexy, we thought. This might have been the attraction when we took that first puff. How different our perception is now. We have changed, and our growth is significant. As smokers, there was little we could do — whether reading, conversing, driving, or simply kicking back — without a cigarette as a crutch. Now we know the laughter and good times, the quiet, romantic moments, or the problem-solving situations are even more rewarding when we're not encumbered by tobacco and its necessary paraphernalia.

Change and growth, like spring and flowers, are paired. And it's good for us to meditate about our positive changes. As humans, we need to feel glory in our growth and be aware that we are moving forward. Our quiet reflection will strengthen our decision and our connection to the inner power that has comforted us throughout the struggle.

I'll take some time today to sit quietly and dwell on who I'm becoming, and I'll be grateful for the growth.

> *"Smoking makes connecting with people difficult."*

We've no doubt come to realize what an intrusion smoking was in our lives. We're particularly aware of this when we're in the company of others who smoke. Their attention to the conversation is frequently fleeting. The search for the elusive book of matches never fails to take precedence.

It's well to remember what it was like for us as smokers. Let's not forget the frantic searches for cigarettes at 2 A.M., the concern over our lack of wind on a tennis court, or the dread of going without cigarettes in no-smoking meetings or in homes bearing the sign "Thank-you for not smoking."

Smoking, like any addiction, can become more important than even the dearest friend. It does ruin lives and relationships, and it sets a poor example for young minds that are so eager to imitate. Isn't it well to have smoking be a thing of our past?

I'll pay special attention to all the times others' cigarettes intrude on my space today, and I'll be glad I've found freedom.

"One of the positive things that happened right away after quitting was the release from fear."

The harmful effects of nicotine have made the news very frequently over the last few years. We've been educated about the danger to our lungs, our hearts, and our circulatory system. Famous people who died from the ravages of cancer have made the nightly news. The less fortunate among us were more personally affected. A friend or relative perhaps died. Even worse, some of us sharing this present struggle are recovering from cancer surgery.

Having quit gives each of us an extended lease on life. And we've been given the manyfolded gift of freedom — freedom from fear that we'll die an awful cancer-ridden death; freedom from an addiction that demanded our time, our money, and our attention; freedom from embarrassment that we couldn't spend time in someone's car or an evening in someone's home or in a favorite restaurant without a nicotine fix at frequent intervals.

I'll reflect on my freedom today and be grateful that I have taken charge of my life.

Day 51

"I still think of tobacco every day even though I'm happier not using it."

Tobacco was a friend, accompanying us everywhere we went. It shouldn't surprise us that we think of our friend perhaps many times throughout a day. When a close friend moves away, we think of her or him often, wishing we could share a triumph or a saddening experience. But we don't have to reach for a phone. We can go to another friend for support or laughter. Likewise, we don't have to reach for a cigarette. We can let the thought slip away and turn our attention to the present.

We're happier not using tobacco because we know we made a wise and healthy decision, and we're empowered by it. Our spirits are strengthened, having quit an activity that oftentimes embarrassed us, frequently impaired our health, and cost us a great deal in money and peace of mind. We may waver at times and momentarily wish for a cigarette — and that's okay. It's impossible to always be happy doing what's in our best interest.

When I think of tobacco today, I'll say a small prayer of gratitude for my decision to not use.

"My self-talk saved me."

We are not victims of the thoughts that crowd our minds. We are in charge of our thoughts, and we can change their content at will — a fact that surprises all too many people. It's familiar to feel powerless over changing our lives, and it's deadly to sidestep our responsibility.

We're the only ones who can change the course of our lives through changing our thoughts. Reprogramming our minds is a simple process. When we replace a negative judgment or an unwanted desire with a quiet mind, a positive feeling or thought will surface — every time. We may have to repeat the process many times over, but that's okay. Negative thinking was repetitive, too.

We can replace the urge to smoke with a quiet mind and gladness that we're able to let the urges pass. In time, this process will be familiar, natural, and spirit-moving.

I am the master of my thoughts. I'll insist on peaceful, helpful ones today.

*"No longer killing myself on an
installment plan feels wonderful."*

When we quit smoking, we also quit deluding
ourselves about the harm nicotine does to the
body. It kills, and our lungs have been damaged.
Time is a healer.

Even though we've been off cigarettes only a
few weeks, a glance in the mirror reveals cleaner
teeth and clearer skin. Our pores are no longer
clogged with the toxins from nicotine. Even our
hair is shinier and less brittle. Nicotine squeezed
life from every part of our body. Time is healing
us.

All we've had to do is stop smoking and every
part of our physical life is adjusting to this freedom from the killing effects of nicotine. But
sometimes we have to personally intervene to
help our attitude adjust. Not every day are we
content without the numbing effects of nicotine.
Some days we fail to appreciate having more energy, cleaner teeth, and healthier skin. Let's look
for support from others who understand our
struggle on the rough days. Tough times will
come — but they will go.

*I'm in charge of my attitude. A moment of
silence will help me adjust it.*

"Quitting was not physically difficult, but quitting any activity that rewards you means losing something from your life."

Grieving is a natural and healthy response when we've experienced a loss, particularly the loss of someone or something that has been dear to us over a long period. Tobacco is such a thing. For all the years we smoked, we were seldom, if ever, more than an arm's reach from a cigarette; we were probably closer to a cigarette than we've even been to a very close friend. We used cigarettes for comfort, to keep us awake, to soothe anxieties, and to signify a breather from a difficult or tedious task. Our excuses to smoke undoubtedly ran into the hundreds.

Giving up cigarettes means we're confronted with hours of activities that have to be handled unaided each day. Of course, we're managing this, and we've been off tobacco for a few weeks now; but the grieving process most likely still lingers. Let's not be concerned. Let's rejoice we are surviving the loss. Let's rest assured that the grief will pass and our satisfaction with being a nonsmoker will escalate. Time is all we need.

Each of these 24 hours ahead of me today will help the grief die and heighten my happiness with being a nonsmoker.

Day 55

"When I was involved in a self-seeking, pleasure-oriented activity like smoking, I was effectively tuned out from the rest of the world."

Very often, conversations failed to keep our attention, and activities like running or tennis were much too demanding of our energy when our focus was on our primary relationship with tobacco. For all the years we've smoked, tobacco was *the* primary relationship in our lives. Sure, we had friends and family whom we loved; but when the body cried for nicotine, we responded regardless of what others needed from us at the moment.

We don't look at our smoking past with a great deal of pride. What we can feel good about is that it is now part of the past. We have charted a new course for ourselves, one that's much healthier and more respectful toward ourselves and our loved ones. No longer does smoking distract us from circumstances and individuals who are in our lives by design. We're free now to more attentively fulfill our role in their lives.

I'm free today to be fully present to all the people and experiences in my life.

"Prior to quitting, if I was upset about something, I would smoke rather than deal with it."

As smokers, we all had so many repressed emotions, and they ate at us, causing both stress and anxiety that clouded most of our waking moments. Because of our smoking, we were unconsciously dishonest with ourselves and with our families and friends. Our feelings were not genuinely felt and shared, which fostered our dishonesty with the people who loved us the most. Relationships are only as strong and healthy as they are open and honest.

As nonsmokers we can look forward to new beginnings with the important people in our lives. The past is gone. We need not lament the shortcomings that plagued us there. The future offers all we need for personal growth, for inner happiness, and for our sense of belonging with the people who surround us. Our future as nonsmokers will be far different from what would have been in store for us had we not so wisely chosen this new path.

This new path I walk today offers me chances I had never dared hope for in years past.

Day 57

"My baby will grow up with a role model who doesn't smoke."

We have all learned from observing others in our lives. Often, in our youth, we painstakingly imitated the behavior and the gestures of people we admired. Our heroes weren't always exemplary role models. Nonetheless, their influence was strong; as our characters developed, we created ourselves in their likeness. How awesome it is to be reminded that we, too, are role models. Others, young and old, may look to us today for the strength to make changes in their lives. Living a smoke-free life-style is a refreshing statement to be making to onlookers. We've needed others to help us make this commitment day after smoke-free day. Perhaps it's our turn now to willingly lend our support and share our strength and hope with someone else.

I'll not forget my responsibility to set a good example today. I may be helping someone when I least expect it.

"I had a million incidences of quitting for two weeks, quitting for three months, quitting for twenty minutes."

Tobacco is a drug, one that we easily got hooked to. To get unhooked takes first a willingness, then a decision, and finally a commitment to experience the pain-filled moments without giving in to the urge to smoke again.

Anytime we've quit and started again, it's only because we gave in to the urge. The urges will always come. But we have the choice to call a friend for support, to reaffirm our decision to not smoke, to recount the benefits gained from not smoking. In the past, we gave in because the urge was stronger than our decision. It was also stronger than our self-love.

This can be the last time I need to quit if that's what I want. The choice is mine alone.

Day 59

"Talking to former smokers and asking them to listen is wonderful support during the hard times."

It is not easy becoming a nonsmoker, particularly a contented one. Some days, some experiences, some ordinary moments will test our resolve to the limit. At times like these, we need the strength and support of others who have survived this experience before us.

And it will help to remember our decision to quit was not a hasty one. We want to be free of tobacco. We don't want to let a 30-second urge take away our freedom, our power over ourselves and who we want to be today or who we want to become tomorrow.

I can call upon friends who understand the intensity of my urge to use tobacco. A sympathetic ear will take away the loneliness of my struggle today.

*"The best thing about not smoking is
it doesn't have any power over me
anymore."*

Today might be a good day to remember how
tied we were to cigarettes or chewing tobacco or
pipes. We should not quickly forget how insanely
we protected our supply — smoking dead butts
in the early morning hours or driving in a blinding storm to the nearest store or gas station because, infuriatingly, we had run out.

How nice it is to get out of bed, free of having
to search for matches. And what fun it is to be
free of needing pockets or purses to carry our
supplies. Newspapers, coffee, and phone conversations are just as stimulating without tobacco.
Thankfully, we've taken back power over our
lives.

*I'll gratefully relish my freedom today, and I'll
appreciate the blessings of being a nonsmoker.*

"I struggled, quitting all alone."

Quitting smoking is still a daily decision for many of us. And it's a decision we must make for ourselves. We've probably tried to quit countless times before — for a spouse, a parent, or our children — and failed at our attempts. We want this attempt to be successful. It's a lonely and individual decision, but we don't have to shoulder the struggle to live with our decision alone. And for that we can be grateful.

To be sure, quitting smoking is a difficult experience, and it's always our choice to struggle through any difficult experience alone. But we have other options. We can look to our inner strength which offers us a partnership strong enough to handle even the most trying circumstance without the aid of a cigarette. And we can look to friends or other men and women who, like us, are developing a new pattern of living, one that doesn't include dependence on nicotine.

I'll seek out other nonsmokers today and get their support if I'm struggling with my decision.

"When I see other people smoke, I'm glad it's not me."

I'm well on my way to becoming a comfortable nonsmoker. I no longer connect smoking with all my routine activities. I've become accustomed to finishing a meal without a cigarette. The beverages I drink can be enjoyed without cigarettes. A drive across town or reading a newspaper doesn't require the companionship of a cigarette. I feel good and strengthened by the choices I've made.

Throughout this day, I'll be mindful of all the times in the past when I would have lit a cigarette. I am not compelled to do it any longer; and I'll willingly share my story with someone else who'd like to travel this road, too.

> *"I really don't want to smoke again.*
> *And I think I'm free."*

When we know we really don't want to smoke again, the major part of our struggle is over. In the past we may have quit to satisfy someone else or perhaps because we knew smoking was detrimental to our health. When we quit for any reason other than we no longer want to smoke, the struggle to smoke again looms powerful. It's important to reflect on how far we've come.

I feel free from my smoking past today, and it's good to recount the advantages of not smoking. My health is improving. I have more energy and lung capacity. My living space is cleaner at home, at work, and in my car, and this benefits me and all who share these spaces. I have more money. I'm no longer self-conscious about finding a place to smoke in public. Best of all, taking back my power rather than letting tobacco continue to rule my life has enhanced my self-worth a hundredfold.

I really don't want to smoke again, and I know I'm free today.

*"I decided early on I wasn't going to
let the weight gain bother me too
much because I think it will adjust
itself over time."*

First things first, and not smoking is the priority. Yet, it's terribly frustrating to struggle with
extra pounds when we're trying so hard to make
a major improvement in our lives. We've come to
know that gaining weight is a common dilemma
for most of us who have chosen this new direction. And dealing with it will one day be our top
priority. But for today, once again, not smoking
is the number one priority.

I've become accustomed to conversations without cigarettes, to car trips with both hands on the
wheel, to sipping coffee and reading newspapers
free from the distraction of billowing smoke and
lost matches. There was a time when most activities were difficult to live through without tobacco as a crutch. But live I did.

*How glad I am that I took the suggestion of
"First Things First."*

> *"Smoking is very much a barrier between people."*

Smoking was a very distracting activity. There was the continual reaching for a cigarette, the unending search for matches or a lighter, and the necessary dumping of dirty, overflowing ashtrays. All of these activities usually occurred in the midst of an important visit with a friend, or a phone call. We simply couldn't give full attention to the friend. Always, to his or her disappointment, our eyes and hands darted here or there looking for the paraphernalia we desperately needed.

And then there was the smoke — clouds of it billowing between our faces, preventing an open, clear vision of each other's face. How hard it is to divulge our inner selves when we can't see our friend's eyes.

Finally, there are the muffled feelings smoking causes, which means we're not being real with the people who love us.

How grateful I am that I've removed the barrier between my loved ones and myself.

"When I realized I could not quit smoking, that I was so addicted it was out of my control and I could not quit, then I was able to stop."

Each of us has had a unique experience with tobacco, how we've used it, and how we got free of it, or struggled to get free. And for none of us has this new identity as a nonsmoker come with total ease. Some of us tricked ourselves into it. Or maybe we bargained with ourselves. Quitting for a spell and then rewarding ourselves with a smoke is common, too.

There is real wisdom in finally admitting our powerlessness over the addiction. When we can do that, we discover a freedom from the compulsion to smoke and also, mysteriously, the personal power to stop and stay stopped.

We can and will become contented nonsmokers. Each day we will experience a greater level of freedom from the compulsion to smoke. And we will understand the subtle difference between quitting and stopping.

Today I will be grateful for stopping smoking.

> *"I had gone through so much in my
> life to be a healthy, strong woman;
> and I didn't want to kill myself with
> cigarettes."*

For many of us, quitting smoking feels like the most difficult thing we've ever survived. And that's a natural reaction. Nicotine is addictive, and the body learned to expect the frequent jolts nicotine promised.

The more years we smoked, the more difficult it is to retrain the body's expectations. But it can be done; we are doing it. Every time we forfeit an urge to smoke, we are supporting a new, much healthier behavior.

In the midst of a craving for nicotine (and cravings will likely haunt us for weeks), we'd do well to remember the many other challenges we've survived. From them we'll gain strength. And from none of them did we die. Divorce, death of a loved one, job loss, separation from family and friends. We've survived — even though we often felt unsure we could. We'll survive this struggle, too. That's the process of human life. Becoming a comfortable nonsmoker is just the next step for all of us reading this book.

I'll try to remember today I'm not alone in my struggle to be a nonsmoker. There are many of us, right now, sharing these same words.

"What I learned was that to become a happy nonsmoker, it helped to think of myself as one."

Our thoughts determine who we are and who we will become. Their power over us, particularly how we feel about ourselves, is awesome. It's very important to remember our thoughts are not given to us by an external source. They are very much our own, created solely by ourselves, which means each of us has the personal power along with the responsibility to decide what thoughts we want to entertain. No thought has the power to dominate our focus without our giving in to it.

Knowing we are responsible for our own thoughts can be both frightening and hopeful — frightening because it forces the issue of taking responsibility, but hopeful because we can choose to be as happy as we make up our minds to be. It is strengthening to understand and accept responsibility for moving our lives in a new, more positive direction. "Life" doesn't simply happen to us. We are co-creators every step of the way.

Every thought I have today is of my own making. I will create strengthening, faith-filled thoughts that will protect me throughout the day.

Day 69

"I can remember walking down the street the first spring after quitting and smelling lilacs before I saw them. That was powerful."

Taking careful note, perhaps even making a list of the positive changes in our physical condition, our attitudes, and our perceptions that have occurred since quitting smoking offers important reinforcement for this decision we have made. The tug to smoke again will happen; as a safety measure to protect us from the urge, we can refer to our list of positive changes.

We need to be grateful for the increased energy we have; the improved self-image; the absence of embarrassment in restaurants because of getting singled out; the regained ability to smell and taste the myriad treats offered throughout a day. It will never be wasted energy to count our new-found blessings as nonsmokers. These blessings are real and earned through hard work and commitment. And these blessings will continue to multiply as do the days of living free of nicotine.

I'll begin my day by counting my blessings, and I'll look for a new one, too.

"Smokers are in prison."

Nicotine used to be in control of our lives. It helped us wake up, we thought. It brought us peace and confidence when we were riddled with anxiety. It smoothed our conversations with strangers. Tobacco was king — it was our god in all matters concerning us. We were at its mercy, bowing to its demands — rifling our pockets and wastebaskets for a lonely cigarette or a smokeable butt, or driving miles in a blinding storm rather than live through the night without the security of a smoke.

The degradation to which we stooped may haunt us. And it's right that we recall those times. Never should we forget the power nicotine wields. We should always remember we're only a puff away from giving tobacco the upper hand once again.

The choice to quit smoking was the right one for us. Let's not ever let the reality of our lives as smokers be clouded by a momentary euphoric recall.

Smoking made me a prisoner in my own home, and car, and skin. My sentence is over!

> *"I realize now I always smelled like
> smoke."*

Few of us realized how offensive the odors
clinging to us were. Our clothes, hair, and breath
quickly labeled us smokers. Our homes and auto-
mobiles were seldom pleasant environments for
nonsmokers. It was as though we were immersed
in an impenetrable and offensive cloud that settled wherever we settled. Not a pretty image. Not
a favorite recollection.

It's exhilarating and refreshing to smell clean.
The stains on our teeth and fingers have disap-
peared. We can detect the smells of spring, summer, fall, or winter wafting through the air. And
we can identify a smoker very quickly.

Let's be grateful we're no longer polluting our
own air, or someone else's.

*I'll breathe deeply today and appreciate my own
good smells and the smells of Mother Nature.*

"My process for stopping began with a decision to stop."

Building a house, writing a book, or taking a course in taxation can be overwhelming if we limit our focus to the end result rather than doing what we need to do one day at a time to get it done. It's the same with becoming a comfortable nonsmoker.

We had to first make the decision to stop smoking. How we will feel on a certain day may not be how we felt the day we quit; even now, in our third month, we still struggle. In time, the urges to smoke will leave altogether, and the memories associated with smoking will no longer be fond recollections.

The early process is tedious, sometimes stirring both anger and depression because we don't want to be obsessed with cigarettes anymore, but we too often are. Being patient with ourselves and others when we're thinking about cigarettes rather than work or play takes extraordinary effort. It's well to remember that no thought forms in our minds without our willing participation. We're in charge. Just by deciding to do so, we can replace any thought with another thought far more to our benefit.

My process is slow; just these 24 hours should concern me, and I can do anything for one day.

"I've come to know that smoking is a screen between people."

Smoking took our attention and offered us something to give our attention to. It was all too easy to divert our emotional energy from the persons laying claim to our presence when we were intent on smoking a cigarette.

Smoke, curling up from our ashtray, blocked our view of another person. The smoke was a subtle yet persistent, physical barrier between two hearts needing to connect.

It's never by chance that we're drawn toward one another; and when we're shielding ourselves with a cloud of smoke, we're interfering with the full measure of growth that's in store for us. The "messenger" is in our midst, and we're only partly in attendance.

There's nothing preventing me from being fully attentive to my loved ones today.

*"I've noticed since I quit smoking I
have much more energy."*

Not all of us care about extra energy for racquetball or touch football, but it's nice and extremely noticeable that we can handle a staircase
with greater ease. We can stroll while conversing
with a friend without getting breathless. Our
lungs will return to an earlier stage of healthi-
ness. This one decision has guaranteed us much
more than greater energy; it promises a fuller,
longer life.

We've no doubt noticed many changes since
giving up cigarettes. The days seem to have more
hours. Our clothes stay cleaner. There's a sheen
to our hair that had not been there for many
years. Food is no longer bland, and the windows
in our cars and homes are free of the yellowish
film that coated them. Far reaching are the
changes wrought by our decision to quit smoking. It was a good decision, one whose impact is
not yet fully felt. The weeks and months ahead
promise additional surprises.

*I'll be grateful for my decision to live longer. I'll
anticipate the future with excitement.*

Day 75

*"The main benefit for me is I expect
to see my kids grow up."*

It's been demonstrated in too many lives that
cigarettes are harmful and often deadly not only
to the smoker, but to those who breathe the
smoker's air. We're not the only beneficiaries of
our decision to quit smoking. Friends, children,
spouses, and co-workers have been given the gift
of cleaner air and the chance for longer lives.

We wonder now how we could have continued
to smoke for so long. We're not dumb people and
yet we ignored the statistics and our common
sense. The addiction is powerful; all addictions
are powerful. The only chance to comfortably
find freedom from an addiction is to turn to
other people, and to the spiritual presence that
resides within us all, for strength and support.
Let's not dwell on the past and question our san-
ity in regard to smoking. Let's look to the present
and rejoice that "then was then and now is now."

*My chances for a longer, healthier life have been
vastly improved by one decision.*

"I sometimes miss cigarettes, even now after all these years."

Having decided to give up cigarettes is no guarantee we won't long for an occasional smoke. It's normal for smoking memories to haunt us. Smoking was there during our celebrations and our traumas. But, now, we don't need to act on a desire to smoke. Each day we experience desires we don't address — perhaps a desire to initiate a conversation with a stranger, order dessert with lunch, or call a lover for a rendezvous. Desires should be acknowledged, but they demand no response.

We can't control the sun, the slow-to-bloom lilac bushes, the newspaper carrier, or the neighbor's dog. In fact, our burdens are few. Our behavior and our attitudes are all we've been assigned to control for this life span. These two assignments make us responsible for our longing to smoke and our happiness about not smoking.

The choice is mine. Will I get on with healthy living and shake the dangerous desires away?

> *"People who smoke are like people not wearing seat belts. It's passive suicide."*

We were probably very content as smokers for a period of time. We liked the comfort, the familiarity, and the absence of loneliness smoking guaranteed. How and when did this contentment change? Perhaps we can no longer recall. It's enough to remember that it did change and we can never go back — at least not to the contentment enjoyed in former years. Now we know too much. Now we know cigarettes were slowly killing us and our loved ones. Now we know each puff drew us closer to the end of our lives.

It's startling to know and hard to accept we were committing suicide on the installment plan. No doubt suicide was the furthest thing from our conscious minds. And yet, suicide was the reality and it is the reality for millions who have yet to join our ranks.

It will bolster our own resolve to share our story — what it was like, what happened, and what it's like now — with a friend whom we suspect also wants to quit making installment payments.

I'll carry my story to someone today and save a life.

*"Tobacco was a friend that I now
know was really an enemy."*

Sometimes through unfortunate experiences, we learned that certain men and women in our lives were not the friends they professed to be. All too frequently, they pretended to be friends to get something from us. Cigarettes got something from us, too — our money, our peace of mind, our healthy bodies, and our souls.

As smokers, we were not acting in concert with our best interests. Cigarettes wielded great power over us, demanding our time and attention, not unlike an inconsiderate person. Perhaps the finest thing we can be grateful for today is that we recognized cigarettes were enemies in disguise, and we assertively took back our power.

It's not difficult to determine who is a genuine friend. Getting quiet within allows our Spirit to share the wisdom. It's that same wisdom that will guide our every act if we'll listen.

*I'll be quiet many times today and just listen
within and find direction and strength.*

> *"If a person smokes a pack a day, and it takes seven minutes to smoke a cigarette, that's 140 minutes a day, almost two-and-one-half hours spent smoking rather than doing something productive. People write books in that amount of time."*

It might have seemed nearly impossible to accomplish anything in the early weeks of quitting cigarettes. We were generally obsessed with smoking memories and the desire for a cigarette. But with the lapse of time, we've grown accustomed to a routine that does not include the customary stops to light a cigarette.

Cigarettes *are* a thing of the past. An occasional urge may surface, but that shouldn't alarm us. Remember, we're in control of our behavior every moment, and the urges will pass.

An unexpected result of giving up cigarettes is we have additional time we can put to good use. Although we often smoked while we worked, we more often stopped working to smoke. Each of us has a list, tucked away in our minds, of things we'd like to do — perhaps take tennis lessons or a painting class or tackle a remodeling project. Now is the time to scratch one thing off the list.

My days are longer now that I'm not spending precious hours in a cloud of smoke. Am I using my time to good advantage?

"I had to stop smoking before I could quit."

None of us have had identical experiences with quitting tobacco. It's valuable to acknowledge there are no right or wrong ways to achieve our goal. It's equally valuable to understand we can learn from one another's experiences.

Sharing our stories about what it was like for us and how and why we quit is a way of helping ourselves stay committed to this undertaking; it's also a way of showing support for someone who's trying to make the decision to take the plunge. It's particularly good for us in this third month of our abstinence to strengthen our personal gratitude for the changes that have occurred since we stopped. Sharing our story guarantees another measure of gratitude.

For some, there's a subtle but important difference between stopping smoking and quitting. Others reprogram themselves to be "born anew" as nonsmokers. The manner of our stopping isn't important. That we do stop is paramount.

An opportunity will come today to tell someone else about my smoking past. I'll take it!

> *"I liked going out in the woods to
> hike, but I realized I couldn't. I
> needed to be near a drugstore."*

Nicotine made prisoners of us. It determined where we could comfortably go and how long we could stay. It demanded our time, attention, money, and a ready supply. We shamelessly sorted through coat pockets, trash, and dirty ashtrays in search of smokeable butts and left children unattended late at night while we rushed to the store for another pack. What a relief to be leaving those days behind.

Nicotine's power is subtle, baffling, and consuming. Until we're very comfortably settled as nonsmokers, we must be vigilant about our behavior around cigarettes. Urges will tempt us, but one cigarette will never be enough.

It's very important in these early months of not smoking to explore new activities and develop new interests. We must refocus our energies in fulfilling ways to reap some meaningful benefits from not smoking — as quickly as possible. Old habits die hard unless new ones take their place.

I'll be open to working on a healthy habit today.

"At frequent intervals, I imaged my-self as a smiling, confident non-smoker."

For men and women from all walks of life and for thousands of reasons, visualization is a technique that has been used successfully — by athletes in preparation for intense sporting events, actors before a performance, and speakers before an important speech. Visualization is a creative form of self-teaching. In our minds we practice our stance or our delivery for when the "real performance" beckons.

It's not immediate that we think of ourselves as nonsmokers; it's sensible to help the process along in whatever ways possible. The use of imagery is simple, successful if practiced, and easily accessible; it can be done in a flash and in any setting — a crowded bus, a busy restaurant, or the quiet of an office or study. We close our eyes and draw our picture — carefully and in detail. We dwell on it, savor it for a moment, and then go on about life.

Our belief in ourselves as nonsmokers will be hastened and strengthened through the power of imagery.

Today I'll use my mind to strengthen my new identity as a nonsmoker as often as possible.

> *"It's so much more comfortable being
> a nonsmoker. There are so many
> places where smoking is discouraged
> — if not flatly prohibited."*

I hated the negative attention I caused because of my smoking. I feared asking for a table in a smoking section when I was dining with non-smoking friends. I feared even more sitting through an entire meal, through all the conversation, waiting without a cigarette. I feared parties in homes where the hosts or hostesses didn't smoke.

I thought I needed to smoke in order to think, to talk, to listen to others. Now I know my need to smoke was my own subtle escape from myself and the situation.

To no longer be imprisoned by the demands of tobacco is like being born again. The freedom we now have can empower us to explore new territories, new activities, new ideas. No longer must we deny ourselves an experience because we have to satisfy a nicotine craving. Our decision to give up tobacco has set us free to fulfill our pride and our goals.

I pray for the willingness to be grateful for my freedom today. It is paving the way for me to grow and change in terribly important ways.

> *"One of the keys of successfully quit-
> ting was I had to quit lying to myself
> about what cigarettes did and did not
> do for me."*

Cigarettes really didn't make us sophisticated,
even though it seemed that way. Nor did they
help us solve problems or make us more articu-
late or creative. And they certainly didn't im-
prove our well-being. However, our delusion
convinced us they did all these things and more.

Tobacco's power was cunning and baffling. It
made our decisions for us. It chose our direction
and defined our goals and limitations. And it
waits in the wings to take charge of us again.

Let's rejoice we've come this far. Gratitude for
our many days as nonsmokers will strengthen us.
We've solved many problems without the
"solace" of a cigarette. We've conversed and been
understood; we've pursued many tasks that we
had mistakenly feared could only be accom-
plished with the help of a cigarette.

*How wrong I was, thinking I needed a cigarette
to achieve a goal. I'm free! What an exhilarating
realization.*

> *"Even now, after ten years, if I were to have one, I know I'd start smoking again."*

Forever, I need to be vigilant over the urge for a single cigarette, even a single puff. For us addicted smokers, there is no such thing as "just one." Many of us had to learn and relearn that lesson many times in the past. Let's not relearn it again today.

Being glad I don't smoke, and wanting just one, is not an unusual circumstance. To get me through a momentary longing, I quietly pray I can remember the benefits that accompany the choice I've made to be free from tobacco. I am healthier. I do smell better. I have more time for friends, personal goals, and fun.

I'll be in charge of my life today. I'll not give my power over to tobacco.

"I'm willing to go through pain if there's a benefit, but with smoking there's no benefit."

It's only because of our delusion that we thought smoking benefited our lives. Certainly, when we started smoking, most of us assumed it made us appear sophisticated, or at least grown-up. At the time, that seemed like a benefit.

Tobacco has turned on us like other drugs do in time. Coughing, colds, chest pains, shortness of breath, stained teeth and fingers; we've experienced all of these during our years of use. But what were the benefits?

It's painful to adjust to life's many turmoils with a mind that's attentive and clear, not focused on the next cigarette. In reality, tobacco has allowed us to escape great leaps of growth we're deserving of by muffling the feelings that would have spurred our forward movements.

As a nonsmoker, I'm giving myself opportunities to grow, opportunities that may not come around again.

Day 87

*"I'm less edgy and less frustrated, and
I'm more effective as a nonsmoker."*

Choosing not to smoke is giving me a sense of
personal power that I didn't have before. I can
make decisions that benefit me! I am in control
of my actions and my attitudes.

For a long time I didn't really want to smoke,
but I did anyway. I felt ashamed, sometimes angry, and preoccupied with it. My preoccupation
often took my attention from people and activities I really cared about. It's easier now to be or-
ganized with my life. I no longer keep
interrupting my chain of thought to search for
cigarettes or matches. The events of the day flow
more smoothly. I'm not in need of the perpetual
"break" to satisfy a craving for nicotine. Being a
nonsmoker has added a rich dimension to the
fabric of my life.

*I know I think better, look better, and smell bet-
ter as a nonsmoker, and the decision to be one is
solely mine, today.*

"I've learned through all of my false starts that coming to terms with being a nonsmoker is really coming to terms with taking responsibility for my health, and changing my identity."

I am personally responsible for who I am, how I behave, what I think, how I feel, and who I become. My attitudes about other people, each situation, and myself are solely manufactured in the confines of my mind. And I will be as happy as I make up my mind to be — about work, relationships, not smoking, and other personal achievements today.

Sensing our personal power is exhilarating. Knowing we're in control of the decision to smoke or not smoke nurtures the inner self. Acting responsibly in the face of all the evidence about the harmful effects of tobacco is like heaping praises on the soul. It's affirming to know we're worthy of life.

My self-respect is heightened each day I choose not to smoke. My ego and my physical body are realizing greater health, too.

"The best thing about not smoking is being free of the control it had over me."

Cigarettes used to control my every action. Before meals, after meals, while driving, talking on the phone, or relaxing, cigarettes were a necessity. What a surprise to discover I can go about my daily activities without relying on cigarettes for companionship or comfort. I can make decisions without a cigarette, and I can go from home to work or to visit a friend without having to check on my supply.

Most of us didn't realize we were prisoners of tobacco, at least not until we had decided to quit. Then it became so very clear. Few of us would ever have allowed another person the breadth of control over us that we so willingly relinquished to cigarettes. How glad we can be that smoking is a thing of the past.

I am my own person now, and I love the challenge of my decisions and the strength bestowed on me as a result.

*"It seems all of us are given the choice
to make the best of our opportunities.
Some of us will."*

Hindsight so clearly details which opportunities we've taken and which ones we've missed. Our progress to date in our work and in our personal lives is a clear indication of our responses toward opportunities. Let's be aware that each moment is rich with opportunity, now as in the past. Our openness and attention to these moments clearly determines how far we'll go.

Presently, through reading this book, we're taking advantage of an opportunity to utilize support for our decision to give up tobacco. For none of us has it been an easy decision every day; but we've made it, and now it's month three.

Many of us have quit before, but our resolve and our willingness are greater this time. We're not struggling alone this time. We're open to the help available from others, from these words, and from the Spirit within. We can be grateful that we've responded well to an opportunity to quit with others rather than in isolation.

I'm not alone. All around people are becoming nonsmokers. I'll say a small prayer for all of us.

AFTERWORD

There's nothing to prevent you from going back to Day 1 and reading once again the messages written especially for you — the new non-smoker. Most of us continue to need support and comfort; a second reading of all or some of the meditations will offer strength as well as solace.

Many people throughout the world rely on the ongoing support that daily meditations provide. Those of us in search of continuing personal growth realize that we're always "becoming" — that the adventure never ends. And we specifically discover that the growth we attain allows us to see anew the many subtle meanings inherent on each page of every meditation book. The more we grow, the more we can see possibilities for even further growth.

So do not feel that this book can offer you nothing more. Its job, perhaps, has only just begun. Treat its messages as friends who will never abandon you, but who will comfort you in the days and months ahead.

INDEX

A

Acceptance of nicotine addiction, 76-77
Acupuncture as quitting technique, 41, 82, 154
Adulthood, smoking as symbol of, 112
Aerobics, as Higher Power, 18, 21
Affirmations of strength, 201
Alcoholics Anonymous, as support for nonsmoking, 76, 80, 97-98
Alcoholism, smoking and, 34-35, 56-57, 115
American Cancer Society no-smoking clinics, 103
Anger, quitting and, 5-6, 117-118
Anti-smoking gum, 154
Asthmatics, smoking around, 89
Aversion therapy, 82

B

Behavior modification as quitting device, 19, 184-185
Behavior patterns, changing, 99-100
Benefits of nonsmoking, 42-43, 80-81, 149-150
Brain, nicotine stimulation of, 12-13
Brown cigarettes, 104

C

Cancer, fear of as quitting incentive, 17, 149, 153, 175-178
Carrot sticks for oral fixation, 101
Chemical dependency, smoking and, 105
Chewing tobacco, 113-114, 118, 120

V

W

Other titles that will interest you . . .

Twelve Steps for Tobacco Users
For Recovering People Addicted to Nicotine
  by Jeanne E.
  A recovering smoker shares her interpretation of the Twelve Steps that, applied to nicotine addiction, helped her stop smoking. This booklet can help you take a fresh, new breath from life—caring guidance for about the cost of a pack of cigarettes. (25 pp.)
Order No. 1419

The Promise of a New Day
  by Karen Casey and Martha Vanceburg
  Healthy living—making the most of each moment, each day, each experience—is the heart of this daily meditation guide that reaches out to all of us who seek changes and depth in our lives. (400 pp.)
Order No. 1045

Worthy of Love
Meditations on Loving Others and Ourselves
  by Karen Casey
  A collection of weekly meditations exploring the challenge of love. *Worthy of Love* is a celebration of life for all of us who have struggled to learn to express, and to accept, love. (106 pp.)
Order No. 5005
